Demystifying
Anorexia Nervosa

Developmental Perspectives in Psychiatry

SERIES EDITOR
James C. Harris, M.D., Johns Hopkins University

Tuberous Sclerosis Complex, 3rd Edition
Manuel Rodríguez Gómez, M.D.
Julian R. Sampson, D.M.
Vicky Holets Whittemore, Ph.D.

Neurodevelopmental Disorders: Recognition and Treatment
Randi Hagerman, M.D.

Demystifying Anorexia Nervosa:
An Optimistic Guide to Understanding and Healing
Alexander R. Lucas, M.D.

Demystifying
Anorexia Nervosa

An Optimistic Guide to Understanding and Healing

Alexander R. Lucas, M.D.

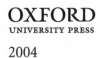

OXFORD
UNIVERSITY PRESS

2004

OXFORD
UNIVERSITY PRESS

Oxford   New York

Auckland   Bangkok   Buenos Aires   Cape Town   Chennai
Dar es Salaam   Delhi   Hong Kong   Istanbul   Karachi   Kolkata
Kuala Lumpur   Madrid   Melbourne   Mexico City   Mumbai   Nairobi
Sao Paulo   Shanghai   Taipei   Tokyo   Toronto

Copyright © 2004 by Alexander R. Lucas, M.D.

Published by Oxford University Press, Inc.
198 Madison Avenue, New York, New York 10016

www.oup.com

Library of Congress Cataloging-in-Publication Data
Lucas, Alexander R., 1931–
  Demystifying anorexia nervosa : An optimistic guide to understanding and healing / Alexander R. Lucas.
    p. cm.
  ISBN 0-19-513338-2
  1. Anorexia nervosa—Popular works. I. Title.

  RC552.A5L83 2004
  616.85'262—dc22   2003015460

9 8 7 6 5 4 3 2 1
Printed in the United States of America
on acid-free paper

To my patients

CONTENTS

In the entranceway of my home hangs a bas relief showing the head and shoulders of a thin young woman carved from a piece of walnut by Eduard Dietmaier. Her face and long neck are hauntingly beautiful but her eyes are pensive and sad. They suggest the sadness that typifies the many faces of anorexia nervosa. The carving's beauty has a magical appeal but masks the suffering beneath the surface. So it is with the girls and young women who suffer from anorexia nervosa. Their outward thinness at first draws envy from their peers, calls forth compliments from their friends and family members, and is a visible badge of their ability to deprive themselves. But inside their bodies grows a malady that can be as relentless and destructive as cancer. Often it is as difficult to heal, and sometimes it leads as inexorably to death.

Thousands of articles on anorexia nervosa have been written in scientific journals since 1868. Hundreds of books have appeared. Yet there is still much ignorance and confusion about the disorder. In the latter decades of the twentieth century the overwhelming number of feature articles that appeared in newspapers and popular magazines, and the many televisions shows about eating disorders, created public awareness but also perpetuated false notions and myths about these disorders. The scientific articles included individual case reports, studies of small and large series of patients, studies of the frequency of the disorder in populations, studies of the causes and vulnerabilities, reports of the effectiveness of various treatments, and studies of the outcome of the disease. These articles are of interest primarily to professionals working in the field. The average person, wishing to learn more about the disease, has difficulty knowing where to turn because there is such a mass of information available. Assimilating this information is difficult enough for the professional familiar with the subject, but it must be arduous for the intelligent lay person. Sources of information can be found in a public library or large bookstore, in a research library, and increasingly on the Internet. Sifting the wheat from the chaff, and facts from myth, becomes a formidable task. When one is exploring the subject for a high school science project or college research paper the challenge can be intellectually stimulating. The stakes are much higher, however, when seeking information in order to understand a family member afflicted with the disorder. When parents of a teenager with the disorder are trying to learn about the disease, the reliability of the information becomes a critical, even life or death matter.

For more than a century anorexia nervosa has been a puzzling disorder. Writers have asked, "How could people afflicted seemingly 'choose' not to eat, and how might not eating become a central obsession?"[1] Eating is such a fundamental biological process necessary to life that families and friends are left perplexed when a young girl starves herself. The irony is that she most often does not intend to starve herself or want to die, but to the contrary, she wants to become a better, more noble, and more attractive person. Those who become anorexic typically have the qualities of being persistent and tenacious in their strivings. They achieve superb control over eating but lose control over other aspects of their lives.

My aim in writing this book is to demystify the disease and to provide a practical guide for parents who are faced with a seemingly insoluble situation. I have tried to provide reliable information about the disease in a straightforward way. I give a broad overview of the condition and a context from which the reader will better be able to evaluate other sources of information. I hope to convey a sense of perspective gained from experience. Thus, the book is a highly personal one. During 40 years of work as a physician specializing in child and adolescent psychiatry I evaluated and treated hundreds of patients with anorexia nervosa as well as many with other eating disorders.

Those with eating disorders included not only youngsters but also many adults. I came to know their thoughts, motivations, and aspirations. I had the opportunity to study the physiological and nutritional aspects of the disorder and the epidemiology of eating disorders. That research gave me the opportunity to examine the medical charts of thousands of individuals, whose records went back as far as the beginning of the twentieth century. This experience, gained first while working in the State of Michigan Department of Mental Health and later in the large multispecialty medical center at the Mayo Clinic in Rochester, Minnesota, gave me the opportunity to appreciate the great diversity with which the disorder presents itself. Patients who develop anorexia nervosa differ one from another and there is a broad spectrum of severity.

In order to make the text vivid, case histories are presented as examples of the varied forms that eating disorders can take. In these stories, names and identifying information were changed. This was done to protect the confidentiality of the real people who were treated. Some of the cases are composites to illustrate certain points. I did not include highly personal details of people's lives that might make them identifiable. The pronoun "she" is mostly used to refer to patients because the overwhelming number—9 out of 10 anorexics—are female.

I have learned that patients with anorexia nervosa grow up in diverse family situations. Many pathways lead to the disorder. The generalizations and stereotypes portrayed in popular articles do not exist for most of the real persons with the disease. A wide range of personalities and temperaments exist among the individuals who develop anorexia nervosa. Once the disease is established, however, the effects of starvation have a powerful effect, making patients behave and appear alike. Families understandably react to a starving daughter and her unusual behavior with heightened concerns and distress. These concerns are reinforced because the most severe cases and those with the worst outcomes have often received the most publicity.

The book is directed chiefly to the families of anorexic patients and to others who want to become more informed about the disorder. The case histories present insight into what it is like to have the disorder and provide some clues as to why capable young girls and boys would engage in such damaging behaviors. Throughout the book I have maintained a tone of optimism and hopefulness. This is warranted because most individuals who develop anorexia nervosa will recover and lead normal, happy, and productive lives. While the recovery process takes time, families can be hopeful about the outcome in most instances.

Rochester, Minnesota, August 1993

ACKNOWLEDGMENTS

First, I owe the inspiration to write this book to James Harris, who suggested that I do so some years ago. I appreciate the confidence that he conveyed and I value his friendship. My teachers in child psychiatry at Hawthorn Center, Ralph Rabinovitch and Sara Dubo, first exposed me to patients with anorexia nervosa and their treatment. It was Dr. Dubo who supervised my treatment of my first patient with anorexia nervosa. She taught me that these patients have a special fragility and need to be treated gently but firmly. I spent the first part of my career at Hawthorn Center and at the Lafayette Clinic in Michigan. When I came to the Mayo Clinic in 1971 my experience broadened. I had the opportunity to meet John Berkman who had devoted much of his career in internal medicine to the study and treatment of patients with anorexia nervosa. He had retired by then but spent many hours with me reminiscing about his patients. The superb medical record system at Mayo gave me the opportunity to study patient records dating from as early as 1916 when Henry Plummer first recognized the disorder among patients at Mayo Clinic. I met Hilde Bruch at a meeting in Denver in 1978, visited her in Houston, and maintained a correspondence with her. Her work strongly influenced my understanding of the disease. My colleagues at Mayo Clinic, notably Jane Duncan, Dick Ferdinande and the nursing staff, particularly Violet Piens, Arla Bernard, and Shari Brumm, played a major role in developing our inpatient treatment program. Additionally, I had the privilege of meeting many colleagues from around the world with interests in eating disorders. Their expertise further contributed to my understanding of these diseases. Among them, Gerald Russell in particular, with his great experience and erudition, was influential. Diane Huse is the dietitian at Mayo with whom I worked for many years. Not only is she very knowledgeable about nutritional issues, but she is uniquely able to relate to anorexic patients and to teach them healthy eating habits. I learned much from her. She contributed the meal plans and made other suggestions in the treatment chapter. Most of all I owe a debt of gratitude to my many patients from whom I learned the most. My editor Joan Bossert at Oxford provided much tangible help and encouragement in preparing the manuscript. She was immeasurably patient and supportive in bringing the book to fruition.

Demystifying
Anorexia Nervosa

CHAPTER ONE

What Is Anorexia Nervosa?

Hilde Bruch called anorexia nervosa a new disease that selectively befalls the young, the rich, and the beautiful. The widespread publicity that revolved around the disease—anorexia nervosa—in the 1970s awakened us to its existence and made it seem that an epidemic had begun. Some anorexic women are indeed rich and beautiful. They were among those that Dr. Bruch described in *The Golden Cage*.[1] More often, though, the illness afflicts teenage girls who come from families of average means. In fact, we now know that it may strike young women of any socioeconomic level. And sometimes even men. Physical beauty is not a prerequisite for becoming anorexic. On the contrary, most anorexic girls consider themselves plain. Some certainly are pretty, but they have no monopoly on beauty. And as for its being a new disease, descriptions of it date from earliest medical history. It was well known to physicians in the latter part of the nineteenth century and throughout the twentieth century. To be sure, it is the third most common chronic illness among teenage girls, but it occurs also in young adult women, and in older ones as well.

Misinformation about the disease abounds and is kept alive by exaggerated media reports. Such reports neither serve the best interest of patients with anorexia nervosa nor do they accurately inform the public. A PBS documentary *Dying to Be Thin* characterized it as the deadliest psychiatric disorder.[2] True enough, it is possible to die of anorexia nervosa, but very few do. Far more teenagers die by suicide due to depression and of gunshot wounds and other forms of violence. Author of *The Beauty Myth*, Naomi Wolf would have us believe that one in five American college women—the best and brightest—are succumbing to anorexia nervosa.[3] She implied that the cause is a societal conspiracy "to keep women down." Further, she cited erroneous statistics claiming that it strikes a million American women every year and that 150,000 of them die. If that were true, anorexia nervosa would be the fourth most frequent cause of death, after heart disease, cancer, and stroke.[4] Facts simply do not support these statements. The historian Joan Jacobs Brumberg, too, in *Fasting Girls*, emphasized the emergence of this disease as a reflection of our culture and described it as a "disease of modernity."[5] Yet she traced the evolution of anorexia nervosa from Victorian times. While she convincingly documented our cultural obsession with thinness, her model of the disease is one-sided and largely ignores its biological aspects.

Anorexia nervosa is not purely a culture-bound illness. It appeared at diverse times in history. As Joan Brumberg acknowledged, it occurred in medieval times as a form of religious asceticism. It occurred before women were emancipated, and it occurs now when women are much more liberated than in the past. It also has occurred in men, who clearly had a different cultural role and identity. There are potent social forces that influence and shape the way people deal with their lives. These social forces influence how illnesses manifest themselves. Yet each individual who develops anorexia nervosa does so in her own unique way. The illness evolves in a complex manner stemming from a woman's own unique biology, her innate personality, and her life experiences. Tolstoy aptly noted that "no disease suffered by a [person] can be known, for every living person has his own peculiarities and always has his own peculiar, personal, novel, complicated disease, unknown to medicine—not a disease of the lungs, liver, skin, heart, nerves, and so on mentioned in medical books, but disease consisting of one of the innumerable combinations of the maladies of those organs."[6]

Thus, each has her own individual disease that only she can have. But even she knows it only partly. Many different circumstances can lead to its beginnings, and many are the ways by which the illness evolves. Yet often the beginnings are obscure or lost to memory. Others may see the external changes of anorexia nervosa in another, but the sufferer may remain oblivious to the onslaught of the disease and the concerns of family and friends. Once the starvation process has advanced beyond a critical point, the disease becomes relentless and tenacious. In turn, the illness itself affects her biology and her environment. Starvation causes profound physical changes that affect growth, maturation, and emotions. The gradual wasting of the body and associated behavioral changes cause family members to express concern, perplexity, and anger. Family relationships become strained and difficult. These distorted styles of interacting often are mistaken for having caused the problem. More often they are the effect of the illness. Anorexia nervosa is not simply a reaction to cultural pressures and expectations; nor is it caused by family discord.

Writers throughout the past century have ascribed to anorexia nervosa an array of causes, from a malfunction of the endocrine glands and faulty child-rearing practices to unconscious fears, perfectionistic strivings, or social expectations. None of these explanations is adequate and some are frankly wrong. One or another causal theory was favored at a particular time in history as biological or psychological theories predominated. For some individuals, the explanation can be quite simple, but for others it is complex. The disease does not arise in a vacuum but in a unique person who is growing and developing both physically and psychologically. The disease becomes a process that affects how the body grows and how the mind thinks. Many different events can trigger the onset of the illness in a vulnerable person. Of relevance to each individual is the way in which many factors interact to start the illness, and how they are further influenced by circumstances that perpetuate it.

True to her name, Joy never brought anything but sunshine into her family during the first 13 years of her life. The firstborn to her parents after nine years of marriage, she had been a cherished child. Her father was an ambitious insurance agent in a small Minnesota town and her mother had been teaching high school until Joy's birth. After this long-awaited event, her mother stayed home to care for Joy. They were a happy family, traditional in their lifestyle and values, and actively involved in their community and church. The mother was a tidy housekeeper who scheduled her time well. She liked to dress Joy attractively. The father was well respected in his community. Four years later, a boy was born, and now the family was complete.

Joy herself was a conforming child with a pleasant disposition, rarely showing anger or meanness. She was highly regarded by her teachers, who informed her parents that she lived up to her name. She took her schoolwork seriously in the early grades and was consistently at the top of her class. She began violin lessons, played in the school orchestra, and practiced diligently without having to be reminded. She also participated in soccer and in swimming. In junior high school her schedule became filled with practice, club participation, and her youth group at church.

She had a lifelong girlfriend who began to spend more time with two other classmates in seventh grade, and then turned her interest to boys. Joy wondered why her friend was neglecting her. She recalled a conversation among a group of her friends during which they ridiculed another girl who had "a big butt." Joy began to wonder if she was being shunned because she was getting fat. She scrutinized herself in the mirror and saw with horror that her thighs were bigger than she had noted before. She decided then that she must diet and began cutting out sweets and snacks between meals. Moreover, she had not yet developed more than breast buds and therefore felt inferior to some of her more mature classmates. Despite her early attempts at dieting Joy was not confident that her thighs were getting smaller. She exerted greater effort and eliminated fats and red meat from her meals. Not only did she avoid having her usual snacks with friends and family members, but she promised herself to stop eating before she felt full and to avoid eating at times when she was hungry. These efforts made her feel somewhat better about herself when she stepped on her bathroom scale and noted that she was no longer gaining weight but actually losing pounds. Nonetheless, her friends did not compliment her, and they still seemed too busy with other interests to bother with her. No one even noticed.

At that time she received a "B" on a math test, the first time she had received less than an "A" that year. She was disappointed and angry with herself. She felt that she must be getting "fat and lazy." She was already devoting two to three hours to her homework every evening, but began to study even longer hours and to get up earlier in the morning to do aerobic exercises. Joy became more isolated as she withdrew socially, devoting herself instead to her schoolwork, violin practice, and exercising. She lost six pounds and felt encouraged when her mother complimented her on her appearance. Rather than giving in to her increasing hunger, as most 13-year-olds would at that point, Joy became even more determined and conscientious about her diet and exercise. She took pride in overcoming her hunger, sometimes skipping meals altogether. She began running regularly and took pleasure in the feelings of thirst and exhaustion that she experienced. She tried to see how long she could go without drinking even water and felt a secret joy over her accomplishment. Her dieting gave her a sense of mastery over her body and a certain sense of superiority. She continued to make near-perfect marks in school. Despite all this, she was not more accepted by her peers. Consequently, she believed that she did not measure up. By then she had lost ten pounds. Her cheeks had become somewhat sunken, and her clothes hung loosely on her frame. When spring came and she wore short sleeves, her mother noticed her gauntness and became alarmed. Previously she had just noted that Joy was unusually serious and even irritable at times. It had become apparent that Joy was not eating well at family meals, and then a school counselor had telephoned the mother to inform her that she was skipping her lunches at school. Encouragement and admonitions to eat more had no effect. On the contrary, they seemed to make Joy even more steadfast in her refusal to eat. Mealtimes now became fraught with strife. Joy's father could not understand why she did not want to eat; she was so thin. He became impatient with her and simply told her that she should eat steak and potatoes again without argument. Her mother took a gentler approach, trying to find out what foods Joy would like to eat and cooking separately for her to try to meet her desires. Neither approach led to Joy's eating more and only resulted in arguments between her parents.

By now it was clear. Joy had developed anorexia nervosa in its simplest, typical form. What happened thereafter would determine its outcome and Joy's future life. This would depend largely on her, on the family's reactions, and on the kind of help that Joy would receive.

What is anorexia nervosa? A great many names and definitions have been suggested for it over the centuries. Simply, it is a condition in which an individual, usually a teenaged girl, loses a great deal of weight because she eats less food than it takes to sustain her body's metabolic requirement. The weight loss is great enough to cause undernutrition with impairment of normal bodily functions and rational thinking. It becomes more than the simple dieting that most teenaged girls try. Typically, it occurs in a previously healthy individual. Kelly Bemis, a psychologist now at the University of Hawaii, defined it as well as anyone when she wrote, "Anorexia nervosa is a complex of physical, emotional, and behavioral changes occurring in individuals who starve themselves because of an aversion to food or weight gain."[7] Her definition implies an underlying motivation because of the aversion. The fear of gaining weight or of becoming fat is common. Increasingly, though, in recent years, such a fear is not expressed, and no conscious motivation for the behavior is apparent other than the desire to become thinner and healthier.

There are, of course, many other illnesses that cause weight loss. In some of these sufficient intake of nourishment continues, while in others there is loss of appetite and diminished intake. In conditions called malabsorption syndromes and in inflammatory bowel disease the body has lost its ability to absorb food normally. In metabolic disorders such as diabetes mellitus and hyperthyroidism food is metabolized too rapidly and utilized inadequately to maintain normal weight. Consequently, the body breaks down its own fat and muscle tissues to use them for energy. In other conditions, most notably cancer, the body's need for nourishment escalates dramatically because of the proliferating cancer cells that avidly consume the energy generated by the food ingested. These are hypermetabolic conditions in which the rate of food and oxygen consumption is increased.

Loss of appetite occurs with acute infectious illnesses, such as "stomach flu." This results in a person eating less and in temporary weight loss. When the illness is accompanied by nausea and vomiting, more severe weight loss and dehydration occur. Acute illnesses are, as the word implies, short-lived. The infection resolves, and appetite soon returns. There are yet other illnesses in which hunger is diminished. The most common of these is depression. The person with depression eats less because she has lost her appetite, shows diminished interest in food, and loses weight as a result. Unrecognized or untreated, depression may last a long time, resulting in considerable weight loss. In none of the foregoing illnesses other than anorexia nervosa is there motivation and desire to lose weight. Weight loss occurs unintentionally.

Innocent dieting is extremely common among teenagers, much

more so in girls than in boys. Usually it leads to only a small amount of weight loss, unless the person dieting is very committed and persistent. Consequently, the weight loss from dieting is usually temporary, and most dieters eventually give in to their hunger. In anorexia nervosa, dieting, often associated with excessive exercise, is persistent and continues beyond what is reasonable. It differs from other illnesses involving weight loss because the body remains healthy for a time, is able to absorb food, and is able to metabolize it normally. The anorexic person feels hungry, at least at the beginning, when she is making great efforts to cut back on what she eats.

Simply put, anorexia nervosa involves substantial weight loss in a previously healthy person because of inadequate nourishment over a long period of time. When an adolescent girl who is about average in height and weight loses a considerable amount of weight—say 15 percent or so below her normal weight—her menstrual periods will stop. The girl with anorexia nervosa typically believes she was getting fat, and still sees herself as being fat even after she has lost some weight. By the time she has lost sufficient superficial body fat and weight to be taken to see a physician, she may persist in this belief and be overconcerned with her body. She may then misinterpret the appearance of her loose skin as flabbiness and fat.

Anorexia nervosa has been known for several centuries, but chiefly in the past 30 years have special efforts been made by the medical profession to describe specific criteria for its diagnosis. This was part of the effort in the field of psychiatry to document objective criteria for diagnosing mental disorders. Unlike many physical illnesses, in which a laboratory test may confirm the diagnosis, the diagnosis of most psychiatric disorders has depended on the identification of certain symptoms the patient feels or on behaviors that others can observe. This is particularly true for anorexia nervosa. Despite our rapidly advancing medical technology, diagnosing anorexia nervosa still depends largely on the story that is elicited from the patient and from her physical appearance. There are no laboratory tests or biological markers that confirm its presence.

Anorexia nervosa has come to be included among the mental disorders largely because psychiatrists have diagnosed and treated patients with the disorder. This has had the unfortunate consequence of overemphasizing its emotional components. In reality, anorexia nervosa is as much a physical disorder as it is a psychiatric one, and certainly the long-term consequences and complications affect the physical health of the individual. Regardless of the wisdom or accuracy of including anorexia nervosa among psychiatric disorders, the disorder and its definition have become established in the psychiatric nomenclature. An unfortunate consequence of this labeling has been the preclusion of insurance benefits for anorexic patients in policies that exclude or limit psychiatric benefits.

In subsequent chapters I will show how anorexia nervosa evolves, how it is diagnosed, how it is treated, and what its outcome is. Its understanding in the medical literature was based on the study of very sick patients who have been in hospitals and those disturbed enough to see psychiatrists. Publicity was accorded to dramatic cases of extreme emaciation, among which there have been some individuals who died. There are many causes and reasons for a person to become anorexic. The cause cannot simply be traced to body chemistry, innate temperament, family constellation, life experiences, or society. For most who are afflicted, multiple factors interact in complex ways to determine how the disease is manifested. And there is much diversity and variability among those who develop the disease. Some individuals are vulnerable in ways that are still not fully understood. Fortunately, most girls and boys in our society do not have it in themselves to become anorexic. Yet they are exposed to the same circumstances as those who do. Without certain vulnerabilities most girls do not become anorexic despite being exposed to circumstances that lead to the disease in others. Different characteristics in the makeup of the individual and her life experiences lead to the onset of the disorder. Patients with anorexia nervosa look and behave remarkably alike during the illness because of its profound starvation effects, but they arrive at their illness in diverse ways. Moreover, they follow different paths as they recover, remain ill, or respond to treatment. Most typically the illness happens at some time during puberty. That causes the pubertal process to be stalled. For recovery to occur, the stages of pubertal and adolescent development must be revived and successfully completed.

How, then, does the illness evolve? In the next chapter we will learn more about how this process unfolded for Joy and for another young teenager, Andrea.

CHAPTER TWO

How Does Anorexia Nervosa Evolve?

Anorexia nervosa arises in ordinary families like yours and mine. It does not require extraordinary circumstances. It can strike when least expected. Most parents of anorexic patients have raised their children admirably. Rather than conforming to a particular style of parenting, they have used a variety of parenting styles. They have not necessarily been overcontrolling as some of the literature would imply. Blaming parents for causing the disease is unjustified. As illustrated in the case of Joy, who at age 13½ was in early puberty, she came from a normal, loving family. Her parents nurtured her, set appropriate expectations, and took pride in her accomplishments. Her behavior was compliant, but not more so than that of many others. She had excelled not only in her schoolwork, but also in music and sports during her elementary school years. She had several close friends with whom she socialized. She was a well-liked participant in class activities and in her other pursuits. She seemed to exhibit more seriousness and greater maturity than her peers, as reflected by her sense of responsibility. Her outward maturity was tempered by some self-doubt. Accustomed to achieving with relatively little effort and excelling in whatever she attempted, she began to expect much of herself. In elementary school she shone in everything she tried and met these challenges quite easily. As she entered junior high school, some of her girlfriends who physically developed more rapidly showed greater interest in boys, who reciprocated their attention. She noted that others had become as good as or better than she at certain academic skills and sports. Others were making more friends and achieving more social recognition. For the first time, she was faced with stiffer competition. Perhaps not surprisingly, she began looking to herself to find reasons for why she was no longer at the top. She was able to perceive minor faults and blemishes in herself and rationalized that she was to blame for being rejected. This triggered her process of self-examination, dieting, exercise, and weight loss.

Another typical evolution of the disorder is illustrated in the case of Andrea. Andrea had always been a shy child, even bashful. She preferred to stay at home with her mother, helping with housekeeping and in the kitchen. She had a few friends, mostly girls younger than she, with whom she shared common interests. She was approaching puberty at age 12½, when she had her first menstrual period. While her mother had explained menstruation to her, Andrea did not ask many questions about it. When it happened, she did not tell her mother and seemed to withdraw more into herself. Her mother thought that the sex education Andrea had in school was troubling her. She had not begun to show the interest in boys that occupied many of her classmates.

She was of average height, at 62 inches. That spring, just after her menarche, she weighed 95 pounds. At the end of the school year, she saw her family physician for a routine examination, and everything seemed fine, although her weight was two pounds less than it had been just two months earlier. Her summer seemed much like any other, but her mother recalled that Andrea probably did not have another menstrual period. At any rate, Andrea did not mention anything to her mother, and the mother found no evidence that she was menstruating.

When school began in the fall Andrea became increasingly withdrawn, even at home, spending much time alone in her room and refusing to interact with the family. In retrospect, the parents recalled that Andrea had begun to skip breakfast and had reduced the size of her school bag lunches to only a half sandwich. Because of her modesty, it had never been her habit to be scantily clad around her siblings or parents, and her weight loss went unnoticed at first. During the late fall and winter she began wearing several layers of clothes, which hid her arms and legs and covered the shrinking size of her torso, but it gradually became evident that she was losing weight. By winter she had begun spending an excessive amount of time in her room, practicing on her flute and cleaning her room repeatedly. She had also begun doing exercises, increasing the time devoted to them from one to two hours daily, often late at night. It surprised her parents that she had become irritable and had begun having temper outbursts. In contrast to her two sisters, she had never given her parents a moment of grief, had never talked back to them, and had been an ideal child. Because of her behavioral changes and apparent weight loss, Andrea's parents arranged for an appointment with their family physician during Christmas vacation. Andrea begged them to cancel the appointment, seeming terrified. She told her mother that she did not like to talk to people but promised to tell her mother what was bothering her. She was bothered by a boy in her class who used profanities and by rowdy kids. She said that she disliked her sisters and people who waste time. She told her mother that she wished she could spend more time with her.

Over Andrea's protests, her parents took her for the examination, realizing that something was wrong. They were startled when the doctor told them that Andrea had lost almost 20 pounds and now weighed only 77 pounds. Despite the weight loss she had continued to grow in stature, and was more than an inch taller than she had been nine months earlier. Other than her weight loss and persistent amenorrhea since her first period, her physician found no medical reason for her emaciation and suspected anorexia nervosa. By the time I saw her in consultation two weeks later, Andrea weighed barely 74 pounds. She sat rigidly upright in her chair, dressed in multiple layers of clothes, and refused to remove her winter jacket in the warm room when invited to do so. Her face was pallid and her face and hands appeared emaciated, showing the outlines of her bones beneath the skin. Her hands were cold and blue.

Although she appeared frightened, when I asked her what was wrong, she firmly said, "Nothing!" I pointed out that there must be a reason for her to be here, and she reluctantly said, "My parents are concerned." "What are they concerned about?" I inquired.

"Doing homework and not watching TV."

"What else?"

"They want me to be with the family like my sisters."

Andrea did not readily enter into the conversation or volunteer any information about her weight loss, but she stoically answered specific questions.

"Why have you lost weight?"

"I'm kinda scared to eat."

"Why?"

"I'm afraid I'll look fat if I eat."

"How do you look?"

"I don't know."

"How do you think you look?"

"Depends."

"Depends on what?"

"I'm not sure how I look."

"How do you feel?"

"Well, sometimes I feel really tired but like I really need to keep going. Sometimes I have headaches all the time. Sometimes like I'm lost and things could be better. I never used to talk to my Mom. I'm cold all the time."

I again asked her, "How do you think you look now?"

"Compared to other girls—a little bit thin. Before Christmas I used to exercise really a lot—a couple of hours a night. Then I got really mad. If I don't do my best I might become rotten and couldn't carry out my goals. I used to have goals of exercising. Now my Mom told me I didn't have to do so much."

"What other goals do you have?"

"To say my prayers at night. I used to stand to pray, but now I can get into bed where it's warm. I used to have to include everyone and everyone's problems."

"Are there other things you're worried about?"

"I'm afraid of getting too big. I'm already as big as my Mom—my bones and my height—bigger than my 18-year-old sister already."

This was the extent to which Andrea was able to describe her fears and her compulsive rituals. I began to see her as an outpatient once a week for a month. She insisted that she didn't want to come, but her parents saw the necessity and brought her each week. She continued to be extremely tense and inhibited, and she worried incessantly about eating and about school. She complained that it was cold at school, particularly in swimming class. Despite her shivering she insisted on participating in swimming until her gym teacher excluded her forcibly. She was encouraged to eat more and increased her intake somewhat, but she was unable to gain any weight. She withdrew even more. One evening her mother found her curled up in her closet, crying hysterically. While she was making an effort to eat more, her eating wasn't producing the desired results. She complained of headaches before and of stomachaches after each meal. It became necessary to admit her to the hospital on a pediatric unit, where her meals could be monitored. Her weight stabilized in the hospital and her mood improved over the next three weeks. She was instructed in a meal plan and for the first time expressed her willingness to eat the necessary quantities. Because she was able to do this she was discharged home and continued to be seen by me together with a dietitian who monitored the meal plan. Andrea became less frightened and was able to gain two pounds in the next two weeks. Although she was now eating adequately, she resisted recording her meals in the food diaries the dietitian had given her. During the next month she became more talkative and spontaneous at home, and was even beginning to reach out to some of her friends. She maintained her quiet demeanor in the interviews and continued to say that she didn't want to come any longer. In another month her weight had increased to just over 86 pounds. She was unwilling to talk about her worries with me but was expressing them to her mother. When she saw a picture of a malnourished child in a newspaper she told her mother that she felt bad because we have too much, while other people all over the world have too little.

Grudgingly she ate the amounts prescribed but balked increasingly at coming to appointments with me. I told her that I would strike a deal with her. If she would continue to gain weight adequately, I would see her less frequently; but if she did not, I would need to see her weekly again. We set a goal of 90 pounds for three weeks. When she returned she weighed 91. In another month her mother reported that Andrea's behavior seemed back to normal. Her weight was above 93 pounds. She was to return in two months, and I kept telephone contact with her mother. Because Andrea was now eating without apparent worry and was again interacting well with her family and friends at school, we stretched the next appointment out to three months. She was continuing to excel in school, making A's in all her subjects, except gym class, in which she had a B. She was no longer studying excessively, was going out for basketball, and tried out for her school play. For the first time she was fighting with her sisters, which both annoyed and pleased her mother. She appeared healthy and robust, weighing 109 pounds, which was near the 50th percentile for her age. Four months later, she was 64½ inches in height and weighed 122 pounds, both of which were at the 60th percentile for a girl now almost 15 years of age. Andrea's menstrual periods had resumed three months earlier when her weight had reached 112 pounds. Andrea had recovered fully from her anorexia nervosa in a relatively short period of time—two years from the onset of her weight loss. She had received outpatient treatment for just over a year.

Andrea displayed both depression and obsessive-compulsive behavior, which was characterized by obsessive thoughts about her appearance and about eating, and she exercised excessively. All of these symptoms resolved remarkably as her nutrition improved. She did not have intensive psychotherapy but rather a supportive approach, which emphasized the resumption of good health and age-appropriate behavior. Initially, when Andrea reluctantly participated in the treatment, I spent considerable time educating her about the physical effects of starvation, explaining the symptoms that she had developed. Whether she really understood or accepted the explanations was difficult to know. At least she seemed to listen. At any rate, my discussions showed her that I was interested in her perceptions and feelings, and they helped us to establish a sense of trust. The treatment included nutritional counseling by a dietitian emphasizing the restoration of healthy eating patterns.

At first Andrea really had no idea why she was not eating. It is quite possible that her fear of eating and of becoming fat was grounded in a fear of growing up. But once she got past the hurdles of eating adequately, gaining weight, and continuing to mature physically, she began coping with the tasks of adolescence. The biological and psychological changes of adolescence were set into motion and there was no way of holding them back. She even began to lose some of her shyness and inhibition, and she joined in the activities of her friends. I had allowed her to make her own decisions about eating while she remained at home. Had she been forced to eat, her resistance to treatment would

have heightened. Andrea was fortunate to be able to respond to the biological drive of growing up. Others tenaciously hold on to their desire
to be thin and require more intensive psychotherapy. Still other patients
require much longer periods of hospitalization in order to recover.

Work with her parents focused on helping them to cope better with
Andrea's illness and on assuring them that they were not at fault. Andrea basically had a very satisfactory relationship with her parents. She
was much more dependent on her mother than most 14-year-olds, but
as her illness improved, this dependence lessened. She was later than
most of her classmates in seeking adolescent independence. Part of
this delay was due to her illness, and part of it was due to her inherent
temperament.

Lori Gottlieb, in *Stick Figure*, described her thoughts and experiences as
an 11½-year-old growing up in Beverly Hills, based on the diaries that
she kept at the time.[1] Now a 30-year-old medical student at Stanford
University, she was a precocious preteenager when she wrote her diaries.
Her mother and the adult women she knew exposed her to constant dieting and preoccupation with their appearances. She was bombarded
with the message that women eat less than men and boys. Her father
and brother always were encouraged to eat more. The discussions
among her friends and the magazines she read gave her the message that
she should look sexy. That meant having breasts, but to be thin. Certainly not to have thunder thighs. She discovered that her butt was bigger than her popular cousin's, and then she became weight conscious
when her cousin revealed her weight. Lori began reading diet books but
was frustrated by learning that each book had different rules. The one
thing they had in common was that a person had to be very committed
to lose weight. Neither the highly emotional expressions of her mother
nor the rational comments of her father were helpful in dissuading her
from her goal: "I was thinking that I'd wish to be the thinnest girl at
school, or maybe even the thinnest 11-year-old on the entire planet."
Inevitably, conflicts with her parents ensued over her eating.

Lori's dieting brought her to her pediatrician and eventually to a
psychiatrist. She protested that her parents were making a big deal over
nothing. She was just trying to eat healthily. Eventually, she was hospitalized but persisted in fighting the efforts to make her fat. Her book is

valuable and unusual in describing her thoughts and feelings and revealing great self-insight.

One doesn't have to grow up in Beverly Hills among stars and starlets to develop anorexia nervosa. Young girls growing up on farms in Iowa and in small towns in Minnesota are exposed to similar media influences, and they acquire many of the same thoughts and ideas that Lori did. They read the same magazines and view the same images of thin models and emaciated waifs in brand-name underwear. The individual manifestations may differ, but their goals are the same—to be the best at dieting. Local influences may color the way in which food restriction is carried out. A girl living on a farm in Iowa refused to eat corn. She rationalized that corn was fed to calves to make them fat, and she was not about to become a fat cow.

Most typically, a high school girl who had been a valued and conforming child faces the biological and social challenges of adolescence and doesn't believe she measures up. Her expectations have been for perfection in all of her pursuits. As illustrated in Andrea's case, often she had excelled in many areas during her elementary school years. Her academic grades have been at the highest level because of her conscientious hard work. She played a musical instrument and practiced diligently. She participated in a sport and worked at it. And she had been active in clubs, church, and other activities. In elementary school she shone in all of these tasks and carried them off easily. As she entered junior high school or high school, she became more challenged in one or more areas. She noted that other people were as good as or better at some of them than she. That made her study harder and work harder at her lessons and activities. Moreover, she may have found that others were making more friends and were achieving more social recognition. Perhaps not surprisingly, she began looking to herself to find reasons for why she was no longer among the most popular girls. Did she need to study harder and for longer hours? Was there something wrong with the way she looked? Was she getting too fat and lazy? There might be an event that would confirm her fears: an undesirable test grade, a slight from her best friend, a comment that her hips are becoming heavy or that her stomach is too big. This is how the stage is often set for a girl to begin dieting. It may begin quite innocently and unnoticed. She may also begin exercising more and more. A whole host of situations may trigger the process that leads to the disease. Many variations in any number of scenarios may play themselves out, depending on the circumstances in a particular girl's life. The common thread in the process is the inexorable weight loss. Once it reaches a critical point, characteristic physiological and psychological changes take place that define and perpetuate anorexia nervosa.

CHAPTER THREE

How Common Is Anorexia Nervosa?

Just how common is anorexia nervosa? The answer depends on how we define the disorder. In other words, how much deviation in eating behavior, distorted thinking about one's body, and physical effects of inadequate diet are necessary to qualify as anorexia nervosa? I believe, as does George Hsu, that dieting and anorexia nervosa are on a continuum; therefore the point at which harmless dieting ends and anorexia nervosa begins is arbitrary.[1] Dr. Hsu is a psychiatrist at the New England Medical Center and Tufts Medical School in Boston. Studies that have asked individuals to rate themselves with regard to attitudes about eating and body image and about dieting behaviors have come up with very high rates of concern about eating and body image among females and somewhat lower rates among males. In some studies, almost half of college women surveyed expressed "abnormal" attitudes. To my mind, this does not represent anorexia nervosa, nor does it represent an eating disorder. Rather, it reflects common societal attitudes about eating and self-concept. For anorexia nervosa to occur, physiological and psychological function must be impaired. The criteria for its diagnosis must be clearly defined. The best ones we have are those defined in the *Diagnostic and Statistical Manual of Mental Disorders* published by the American Psychiatric Association.[2] These criteria are imperfect, but are the best available. They are now generally accepted throughout the world and are used in most research studies. Diagnosis of anorexia nervosa is discussed more fully in Chapter 8. Accurate diagnosis is nec-

essary for epidemiological studies. An aim of epidemiology is to determine the number of cases of a disease in a population. Broader or narrower definitions of the disease will yield more or fewer cases.

Anorexia nervosa once was thought to be very rare but is now quite
common. It is, in fact, the third most common chronic disease among
teenage girls. In the distant past it often was unrecognized for what it
was. Therefore, reports in the medical literature were limited, creating
the impression of rarity. Not until the 1960s did anyone try to determine the frequency of the disorder in the population. Sten Theander,
at the University of Lund in southwestern Sweden, studied the medical
records of women who had been treated for anorexia nervosa between
1931 and 1960.[3] From these records he estimated the frequency of the
disorder in the surrounding population, assuming that the patients
had come from the region served by the hospital. Theander found an
increase in the numbers during that time, but cautioned that the increase might be more apparent than real because of better identification of the disorder. Other studies, in northeast Scotland and in Monroe County, New York, also suggested increases over time.[4,5,6,7] The
incidence figures for new cases per year rose from less than one per
100,000 individuals before 1960 to 4 per 100,000 individuals in 1980.
These studies were based on psychiatric case registers, rosters of individuals who had been seen by psychiatrists in those communities. A
study in Zurich, Switzerland, counted patients who had been hospitalized.[8] The investigators of all these studies assumed that the patients
came from the surrounding regions and based their calculations on the
populations of those areas. Thus, the patients were not drawn from a
defined geographic area, and the results represented estimates of incidence. Additionally, a requirement of the studies was that the patients
had received treatment for their disorder either in a hospital or by a
psychiatrist. Individuals in the surrounding communities who were
treated by nonpsychiatric physicians and those who had received no
hospital treatment would not have been included.

In my own studies in Rochester, Minnesota, my colleagues and I used
a different methodology and produced quite different results.[9,10,11] We
studied the medical records of all individuals residing in the community of Rochester who could possibly have had anorexia nervosa. We
did this by reviewing many thousands of records of women and men

who had weight loss from any cause, and of women who had menstrual irregularities. The time span we studied was considerable: from 1935 through 1989. We applied standard criteria for diagnosing the disorder to the information gleaned from the medical records and identified individuals who had definite, probable, and possible anorexia nervosa. Thus, we came up with numerous individuals who had never been formally diagnosed with anorexia nervosa but who had all the characteristics of the disorder that are now recognized. Most of these people had never been hospitalized for the disorder, and many had never seen a psychiatrist. Thus, they would have been lost to a study that depended on hospital records or psychiatric case registers. Some earlier diagnostic criteria had set an upper age limit at 25 years. We used no age limits in searching for these individuals. Thus, we identified persons in the community from a broad age range. The youngest girl was 10 and the oldest woman was 59 when her disorder began. As expected, however, by far the largest numbers were girls and women between the ages of 15 and 24 years; one in 10 subjects was male (see Figure 1). To our surprise, for

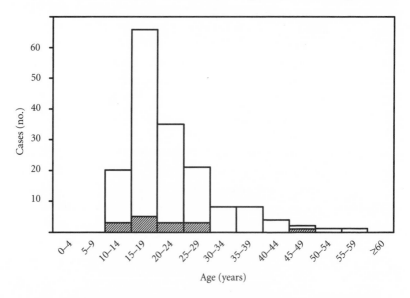

Figure 1. Distribution of age at diagnosis of anorexia nervosa. Females, open bars; males, cross-hatched. Adapted from Lucas, AR, et al. 50-year trends in the incidence of anorexia nervosa in Rochester, Minn.: a population-based study, Am J Psychiat 1991; 148:917.

the entire age group, females and males together, we found no remark-able increase over time. In the typical age group, however—the females between 15 and 24 years of age—there was a significant increase from 1935 through 1989. The occurrence of anorexia nervosa in older women had remained the same over time, and the occurrence in males had also remained constant (see Figures 2 and 3).

We found the overall incidence rate (new cases occurring per year) to be 8.3 per 100,000 persons in the population. For females it was 15.0 per 100,000, and for males it was 1.5 per 100,000. Among 15- through 24-year-old females it rose from about 15 per 100,000 in 1935 to about 60 per 100,000 in 1989.

Our study showed higher incidence figures than other studies be-cause we screened the entire community, regardless of whether the subjects had previously been diagnosed or treated. The incidence fig-ures derived by Hoek and Brook, who surveyed general medical practi-tioners in Holland for possible cases of anorexia nervosa, came closest to ours.[12]

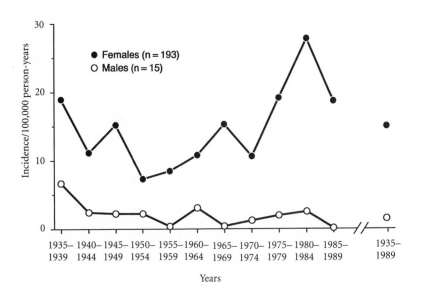

Figure 2. Incidence rates for anorexia nervosa in residents of Rochester, Minnesota, 1935–1989. From Lucas, AR, et al., The ups and downs of anor-exia nervosa, Int J Eat Disord, 1999; 26:401.

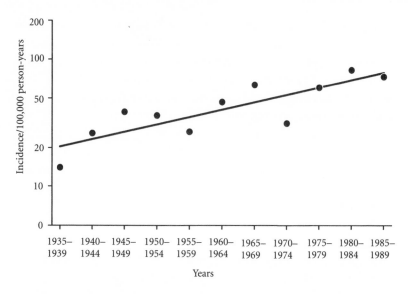

Figure 3. Incidence rates for anorexia nervosa in 15 to 24-year old female residents of Rochester, Minnesota, 1935–1989. From Lucas, AR, et al., The ups and downs of anorexia nervosa, Int J Eat Disord, 1999; 26:402

Clearly, among teenage girls and young women, the disorder is much more frequent now than it was in the past. We found the prevalence of the disorder (number of cases in the community at any given time) to be about 1 in 200 older teenage girls. This figure is almost identical to that found by Råstam in Göteborg, Sweden, among all 15-year-old schoolgirls,[13] and it is the same as the prevalence found in a 1976 study by Crisp, Palmer, and Kalucy in London, where they surveyed girls in nine different schools.[14]

Formal studies of incidence and prevalence have been done in New York State, in Minnesota, and in several western European countries. It is likely that the rates for anorexia nervosa are similar throughout North America and Europe. In South America, particularly in Brazil and Argentina, the disorder is not uncommon. Reports of many cases have come from Australia and New Zealand as well. The evidence suggests that anorexia nervosa evolved primarily in "Western" cultures, but as interest in the disorder has grown, more reports have come from elsewhere in the world. It is said that the disorder has become more frequent in Japan. Young women in countries that have become westernized seem to be similarly vulnerable. Increasing globalization and the homogenization of cultures worldwide have hastened the spread of the disorder. In contrast, it is still rare in the Middle East, with the exception of Israel. It is nearly unheard of in Africa except in South Africa and Egypt. Although there are some case reports of anorexia nervosa in African American women, most of the reports are not of typical anorexia nervosa. The disorder is still very rare in this ethnic group.

What makes for the differences in prevalence among different cultural and ethnic groups? First, the disorder is more frequently recognized in developed countries that have sophisticated medical care than in those countries with more primitive medical care systems. Second, the attitudes toward body shape and dieting differ among cultures. Western European and North American cultures place high value on slimness in women whereas Middle Eastern, African, and Polynesian cultures value adiposity. In such cultures anorexia nervosa is unlikely to occur. But there must be other factors. Starvation occurs with great frequency in underdeveloped countries. Starving individuals develop physical effects resembling the starvation effects that are seen in anorexia nervosa, yet they don't have the disorder. The difference is that they don't want to starve. When food becomes available they will eat eagerly, despite the physical discomfort that comes from distending a shrunken stomach. They may even gorge themselves when given enough food to do so. On an episode of the TV show *Survivor* in April 2001, Cody, who with his fellow competitors had been starving in the Australian Outback for many days, won the opportunity to spend a day and night with ranchers on the range. They ate a hearty supper of beef stew and beans. He stuffed himself. Despite being sick throughout the night from overeating, he awakened in the morning and treated himself to a full breakfast including eggs and bacon.

When there is no food, victims of famine continue to starve, and eventually they become indistinguishable from a person with chronic anorexia nervosa who has refused treatment and has given up hope. Knowing the circumstances makes the cause obvious. Another difference is that individuals with anorexia nervosa starve selectively. They make restricted food choices while surrounded by plenty. Their restriction of essential nutrients is not as complete as that imposed on victims of famine. This is why patients with anorexia nervosa do not often develop specific vitamin and mineral deficiencies.

It is quite likely that some individuals and perhaps some ethnic groups have genetically determined protective factors that prevent them from developing the symptoms of anorexia nervosa after dieting. I suspect that this is true for nonwhite populations, among whom anorexia nervosa is rare. Scientific studies have not yet confirmed this hypothesis.

Our incidence figures for the 1980s suggest a leveling off in the frequency of anorexia nervosa. As the century drew to a close, this certainly seemed to be so for the form of the disorder in which adolescent girls strictly curtail their eating without resorting to binge-eating or purging. In its place we have seen more teenage girls and young women who have a mixed symptomatology manifested either by intermittent starving and binge-eating behavior, or binge-eating and purging behaviors known as bulimia nervosa. Our study of the incidence of bulimia nervosa in Rochester showed a sharp rise in incidence among females in the early 1980s (see Figure 4).[15]

After many years of treating and studying patients with anorexia

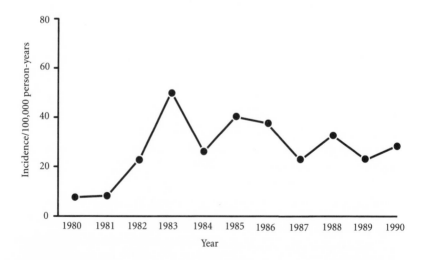

Figure 4. Incidence rates for bulimia nervosa among female residents of Rochester, Minnesota, 1980–1990, adapted from Soundy, TJ, et al., Bulimia nervosa in Rochester, Minnesota from 1980 to 1990, Psychological Med, 1995; 25:1068.

nervosa in London, Gerald Russell identified a new disease in the late 1970s that he called bulimia nervosa.[16] While most of his patients were restricting food and had the typical characteristics of anorexia nervosa, he began to note increasingly that some of the patients were self-inducing vomiting to compensate for episodes of overeating. He noted that they had a morbid fear of becoming fat, much like typical anorexic patients. But they also had intractable urges to overeat, and they avoided the fattening effects of food by vomiting or abusing purgatives. Many of them had a previous episode of anorexia nervosa with weight loss. Russell's long experience led him to believe that the manifestations of eating disorders have changed over time and he found support for this assumption in the scientific literature.[17] Our study and that of Hoek in Holland documented that bulimia nervosa had surpassed anorexia nervosa in frequency by the 1980s.[18] Thus, the form that eating disorders took had changed.

CHAPTER FOUR

What Causes Anorexia Nervosa?

Before her 13th birthday Ynez had been of average height and weight. She weighed 98 pounds. A very pretty brunette with luxuriant, wavy hair, she was the most popular girl in her elementary school because of her outgoing, fun-loving nature. She became infatuated with a boy in her class and wanted to make herself attractive to him. Consequently she spent much time scrutinizing herself in the mirror, brushing her long hair, and noticing small blemishes. The following year she attended a much larger school, housing both the junior high and high school grades. She felt overwhelmed by the prospect of being in this school and she feared failure, even though she was an excellent student. Moreover, she feared that she would not be accepted socially. She strove to become more beautiful, hoping that this would ensure her popularity. As her breasts developed and her hips and thighs grew larger, she became concerned that she was getting fat. Noticing that her waistline was increasing was particularly distressing. She studied fashion magazines and envied the slender appearance of supermodels, comparing her measurements to theirs. She wanted to look like these models. Thus she began to diet and rather quickly was able to lose some weight. Her friends envied her because they failed in their attempts to diet. Ynez persisted even though her friends were baffled because she had never been overweight. Her success at dieting heightened her resolve to continue. Occasionally she gave in to hunger pangs and overate. She tried to vomit unsuccessfully. Eventually she learned to gag herself with a finger. She abhorred the idea of vomiting but it gave her a feeling of control. She could now occasionally eat more because she knew she could rid herself of the food. Her vomiting was followed by mixed feelings of guilt and mastery.

Ynez's weight plummeted to 68 pounds within a year. She had never menstruated. Her hair began falling out in bunches when she brushed it. Her skin became dry and scaly, and her fingers became bluish and cold. Her clavicles and shoulder blades stood out sharply. Her arms and legs became so stick-like that her classmates called her "toothpick." Ynez remained oblivious to these physical changes and persisted in her belief that she was fat. When she pinched the loose skin around her waist she believed it to be fat. She rebuffed her parents' admonitions that she should eat, insisting that she wasn't hungry.

Her father spent long hours at work managing an automobile dealership and her mother taught in the elementary school. When an older brother became involved with street drugs and alcohol, his conflicts with the law occupied the parents' time and energy and distracted them from attending to Ynez. They had hoped that her problem would go away. When it became only too apparent that Ynez was starving herself, her parents finally insisted that she have a medical evaluation. She appeared emaciated and had a slow pulse and low blood pressure. Fine, downy hair had appeared on her back. Because of a heart murmur she was referred to a pediatric specialist for an evaluation. The heart murmur proved to be benign. The remaining findings were all manifestations of starvation. It was noted that there was erosion of her dental enamel from vomiting. The pediatrician then referred her to me for treatment. Ynez seemed motivated for treatment because she understood intellectually that she had carried her dieting too far. She was ready to admit that she felt miserable, being cold all of the time. She tired easily and found it difficult to carry out the many activities she was involved in. Concentrating on her schoolwork had become a problem and she was sleeping poorly.

Ynez was able to increase what she ate, but she was unable to stop vomiting. Thus, after a period of outpatient treatment she required more intensive treatment in the hospital. Her vomiting was controlled in the hospital because her meals were regular, but it recurred after she returned home. Her course was rocky and protracted, with weight fluctuations over the next several years since she was unable to maintain the regular eating habits that were established in the hospital. Periodically she overate. This triggered further vomiting, which had become easier for her to do. Eventually, at age 17 years, her weight reached 106 pounds and she had her first menstrual period. However, she continued to struggle with her disorder into her early twenties.

Kirsten was a rather quiet 14-year-old ninth grader who strove to participate in all the sports at her small rural school. Her older sister was an honor student and a standout basketball player on a team that had consistently been the champions in their league. They had often won their regional competition. That year they were to compete at the state tournament. Kirsten pushed herself to compete athletically with older girls and made the varsity volleyball team, the only one in her class to accomplish this. She rose early each morning to do her schoolwork, and she ran extra miles after school to improve her physical condition. During the winter she participated in basketball but was disappointed not to make the varsity team. It was little consolation to her that the team was among the best in the state, and its members, including her sister, were all eleventh and twelfth grade students.

From August to December she had lost 10 pounds, her weight dropping from 106 to 96 pounds. She had become listless and irritable. Her mother, a bookkeeper at a nursing home, brought Kirsten to her pediatrician in the nearby city. The pediatrician found no illness to account for the weight loss and encouraged Kirsten to eat more, arranging to see her again in a month. By January Kirsten had lost even more weight, now weighing 93 pounds, and she had missed two menstrual periods. A dietitian was called in to review Kirsten's diet history; she determined that she was eating only 500 to 600 calories daily, consisting chiefly of fruits and cereal. Kirsten was selecting foods low in calories, had virtually eliminated fats from her diet, and was skipping her lunches. She insisted that she was eating a healthy diet, pointing out that she had studied the American Heart Association guidelines. What she was unaware of is that her diet was woefully inadequate for a growing, rapidly developing adolescent who was physically very active. She was consuming virtually no fats, very little protein, and the total number of calories in her diet was far below what her body needed.

Her pediatrician continued to encourage her and began seeing her every week. Another month elapsed without progress. Her pediatrician asked me and a dietitian knowledgeable about the treatment of eating disorders to participate in the treatment. It became clear that Kirsten was not heeding her pediatrician's advice and not following her recommendations to increase her food intake. Working closely with the dietitian, I reviewed the situation and spent some time educating Kirsten about her growth and nutritional needs. She had now lost a total of 16 pounds and had missed three menstrual periods. Although eating more, she was exercising excessively. Her hands were cold and blue, the palms of her hands had an orange tint, and her resting pulse rate was 44 beats per minute. She was very tearful, protesting that she had been trying to eat more. I told Kirsten that in order to maintain her health, she must not lose any more weight, and she needed to consume enough food to accomplish that. Since she was expending too much energy, I told her that she could not participate in physical education or in competitive sports for the time being. I warned her that she might need to come into the hospital if things didn't change. Kirsten didn't like to hear any of this but reluctantly listened to her mother, who reinforced my recommendations.

I arranged to see Kirsten again, setting up twice weekly appointments in order to keep very close track of her progress or lack of it. The dietitian would see her once a week. Kirsten was upset about having to miss school for appointments. Her mother nevertheless brought her to the appointments faithfully. Within a week her weight loss had abated. We reduced the frequency of appointments to weekly. Kirsten said little at first, but was willing to go through the motions of following the meal plan prescribed. She knew that she could not participate in sports until she had gained an adequate amount of weight. As we educated her about nutritional principles and the physiological effects of weight loss and weight gain, she began to ask the dietitian questions about foods. She continued to be reluctant to discuss any concerns with me. When I asked her about her schoolwork, her friends, her interest in sports, and her interaction with her sister, her responses usually were brief and matter-of-fact. Some of our conversations focused on the physical changes taking place in her body that resulted from the weight gain. Her fears and anxiety about this process also had to be addressed.

The dietitian and I continued to see Kirsten each week or every other week throughout the summer. Following the dietitian's meal plan, Kirsten gradually accepted greater quantities of food and more variety. Her nutritional state improved as her weight slowly increased.

By the beginning of August, her weight had reached 110 pounds, and by the time school began it was more than 115 pounds. She was now 5 feet 7 inches tall. Kirsten's good progress continued. By the end of the first semester she was achieving A's and A+'s in all of her subjects. She again looked healthy and perky. Her mother said that she had regained her spark. I felt comfortable about having her resume sports, and she again joined the volleyball team during her sophomore year. While Kirsten had been gaining some weight with a period of reduced physical activity through the summer, she would need to eat considerably more to continue gaining weight while actively involved in sports. I pointed out that it is relatively easy to eat enough to maintain weight, but to continue gaining, as was necessary at her age, she would have to push herself to eat more, even after feeling full. Her mother commented that before she was seeing the dietitian and me regularly, Kirsten was encouraged to change her eating habits and was given emotional support, but she had not been given specific guidelines about what to eat. Moreover, no goals had been set for her. We were very specific about what she had to do, emphasizing the seriousness of the situation. Her mother also noted that Kirsten had regained some of her energy and seemed more cheerful around home. She was also beginning to seek out her friends again.

Her participation in volleyball proved to be beneficial. Kirsten ate her prescribed lunches at school. When she came home after practice she seemed genuinely hungry for the first time since the previous winter and ate a substantial dinner. We were able to reduce the frequency of her clinic visits to once every two weeks and later during the school year to once a month. Kirsten participated in basketball during the winter. She remained enthusiastic about her studies and showed renewed interest in her social life. By February of the next year her weight had stabilized at 117 pounds. Altogether the dietitian and I had each seen her a total of 22 times. Her mother kept me apprised of her good progress during her final year of high school. Kirsten had continued to gain a moderate amount of weight and had come into her own socially after her sister graduated from high school and went away to college. Kirsten had developed as a star in her own right, both in volleyball and basketball.

Unlike Ynez, Kirsten was not so much fearful of getting fat as she was driven to compete with her sister and older peers. If she had thoughts about wanting to be thin, she did not reveal them. She placed herself on a reducing diet believing that eliminating fats was the healthy thing to do. Her intentions were good, and she did not realize that she was, in fact, starving herself.

Clinicians have struggled to understand the causes of eating disorders for more than a century, ascribing them variously to biology, psychology, or culture over the years, depending on the currency of the day. One or another of these theories has been favored at any given time. But any such concept of the illness is too simplistic. It ignores history and clinical experience. The latest vogue is to suggest that the cause lies in changes in the body chemistry. Yet ascribing everything to biology alone has as little value as ascribing it all to culture. What's intriguing is how these factors interact to shape the particular signs and symptoms we attribute to the disease.

Although patients with anorexia nervosa look and behave very much alike once their starvation is well advanced, there is no single cause. The antecedents of the illness—the ways it begins —vary enormously. What underlies the problem often may not be discerned at the time of crisis but may come to light much later. Sometimes the precipitant is never known. Dr. Berkman, the internist who treated hundreds of anorexic patients at Mayo from 1930 to 1960, once cautioned me, "Don't ever ask them what caused it, because they don't know."

It has long been recognized that no single specific event or situation causes anorexia nervosa. As with many other illnesses, a combination of vulnerabilities and circumstances is necessary for it to become manifest. In attempting to understand the cause when I was seeing many patients in the 1970s, I tried to develop a working hypothesis to make sense of the disease. It seemed clear to me that quite different circumstances led to the disorder in different individuals. In some, significant life events seemed to trigger the disorder; in many others, there were none. While some families had focused excessively on issues of food and body image, many others had not. In contrast with descriptions in the literature, most of the parents I encountered were not overcontrolling, and they were not excessively enmeshed with their children. While the patients, once they had anorexia nervosa, often had personality characteristics in common with each other, the stories leading up to the beginning of the disorder varied, and the family constellations and parental attitudes differed one from another.

Most children in our society are exposed to similar societal pressures but they do not react alike. It seemed that in order to develop anorexia nervosa one needed to be vulnerable in some special way. Risk factors and vulnerability were not well understood at that time, but clearly some individuals were more susceptible than others. Once the illness began, the patients looked and behaved remarkably alike. They demonstrated profound physical and emotional changes. Their parents understandably became increasingly concerned, and this often led to conflicts. More often than not these conflicts were the result, not the cause, of the illness.

Stimulated by the work of psychiatrist Herbert Weiner,[1] whose conceptualizations of disease process were rooted in the psychobiology of Adolf Meyer, the pioneer of modern American psychiatry at Johns Hopkins University, I proposed a hypothesis for anorexia nervosa that suggested the importance of both biological and psychological factors. I speculated that there was a genetically determined metabolic predisposition that interacted with early life experiences within the family environment. Triggered by pubertal changes, this predisposition could lead to dieting. A vicious circle would ensue, leading to undernutrition, physiological changes, and changes in thinking that constituted anorexia nervosa. In 1977 a psychiatrist, George Engel, working at the University of Rochester, New York, published what was to become a classic paper in *Science*. In it he elaborated the biopsychosocial model of disease. He proposed that all diseases should be viewed within the framework of multiple factors: biological, psychological, and social.[2]

I believed that the influences from these three interacting spheres were necessary precursors of anorexia nervosa and agreed with Engel's model as a likely explanation of the disease. If dieting occurred at the time of pubertal endocrine changes, when girls rapidly acquire body fat, a vicious circle leading to weight loss, undernutrition, and physio-

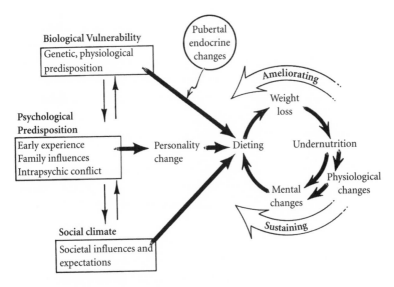

Figure 5. Biopsychosocial model for anorexia nervosa. Adapted from Lucas, AR, Toward the understanding of anorexia nervosa as a disease entity. Mayo Clin Proc, 1981; 56:258.

logical and mental changes would result (see Figure 5). Almost certainly, a biological vulnerability is necessary for an individual to develop anorexia nervosa. In addition, certain psychological characteristics and environmental experiences can reinforce the biological vulnerability, as I further expanded in a theoretical model of the disease.[3]

This interactional model suggests that three factors—biological, psychological, and social—lead to inappropriate dieting at the time of pubertal changes, when girls are rapidly gaining body fat. Each of these three factors has a greater or lesser impact on particular individuals in whom anorexia nervosa develops. Some girls have a strong innate tendency to develop the disorder, but the genetic predisposition must be necessary for the disorder to occur. Most individuals (those who do not have the genetic predisposition) will never develop anorexia nervosa, even though exposed to the same environmental stresses and social pressures that influence vulnerable persons. Many environmental influences reinforce the vulnerability to the disorder and lead to dieting. Certain parent-child relationships are more conducive to the development of the disorder, but in and of themselves they do not cause it. Overemphasis on all aspects of eating, excessive concern by the patient about becoming overweight, and overcontrolling attitudes by parents in a patient's early childhood all have been implicated as contributors. Events as diverse as an illness, a sexual assault, or performance in sports can trigger weight loss and thus play a role in the developing disease. The social climate, where high value is placed on extreme thinness, reinforces any tendency to diet and to lose weight. And overzealous attention to preventive health practices that promote dietary restrictions or exercise also may reinforce this tendency.

Genes

Evidence has accumulated that genetics plays a prominent role in a person's vulnerability to developing an eating disorder, with the risk increasing if there is a family history of eating disorders, depression, or alcohol abuse. Even though researchers believe that there is a genetic influence in anorexia nervosa, the particular genetic link has not been discovered. This connection will have to await results of the ongoing study of the human genome.

Containing at least 30,000 genes, the human genome constitutes the genetic information present in every cell of the body. Individual genes are long sequences of four nitrogenous bases (adenine, cystosine, guanine, and thymine) that make up the double helical structure of DNA. The DNA chains are situated on 23 pairs of chromosomes that are present in the nucleus of every one of the 100 trillion human cells in each body. The function of genes is to produce proteins that have a particular physiological action.

The elucidation of nearly 100 percent of the human genome in 2001 has opened the door to a new world of possibilities. As the genes associated with particular diseases are identified, diagnosis and treatment may be facilitated. However, the practical application of this new knowledge will take time.

Genes responsible for numerous diseases have now been identified. Some diseases are caused by single mutant genes. Examples of these are cystic fibrosis, sickle cell anemia, and phenylketonuria. These can easily be understood and some can be effectively treated. In phenylketonuria the errant gene fails to produce the protein enzyme that metabolizes phenylalanine. The disease is treated by restricting dietary phenylalanine. In the future, genetic engineering may allow the defective gene to be replaced with a healthy one. Other diseases such as Down syndrome (trisomy 21) are the result of the addition or deletion of entire chromosomes. This results in a broad range of physical, developmental, and mental abnormalities. Finally, there are diseases that result from the interaction of multiple genes. These include common diseases such as coronary artery disease, hypertension, and diabetes mellitus, as well as psychiatric disorders. In these diseases the effects of several or many genes interact to create the predisposition to the disease. Environmental triggers then make the disease manifest. This is very likely the way in which anorexia nervosa is caused. Most likely, a number of genes that influence specific physiological and personality characteristics are necessary for anorexia nervosa to develop. The way genes interact to determine personality and temperament is highly complex and poorly understood. The same characteristics that play a role in anorexia nervosa may have beneficial qualities. For example, anorexic patients display a great deal of persistence and compulsivity. These traits may reinforce the illness but the same traits can have a positive influence under other circumstances. Particular genes may enhance or protect against the effects of starvation.

Dean Hamer, chief of gene structure and regulation in the Laboratory of Biochemistry at the National Cancer Institute in Bethesda, Maryland, and Peter Copeland, managing editor of Scripps Howard News Service in Washington, D.C., co-authored the book *Living With Your Genes*. In it they suggested that "anorexia is almost certainly a biological disease that represents a distortion of a natural biological response—the response to famine. . . . The question is not why the behavior starts, but why it doesn't stop. . . . [I]n looking for genes for this puzzling . . . disorder, both genes related to eating, and those involved in emotionality, would be places to start."[4] Because the predisposition for anorexia nervosa undoubtedly involves many genes, both "good" and "bad," treating and preventing the disorder through genetic means will not soon be accomplished.

Just how our genes and environment interact to result in anorexia nervosa is still speculative. It is likely that multiple genes interact to influence behavioral and temperamental characteristics. Genes also are undoubtedly involved in how the body responds to starvation and to treatment interventions. Once we begin to know our genes and mental processses more intimately, these interactions will begin to become clear. Thus, there is no single gene that causes anorexia nervosa, but many genes involved in a dynamic process—the interaction of fundamental biological processes and environment—ultimately resulting in the disease. Genes and environment also determine how each individual responds to her disease. Despite the similarities in starvation effects, each person with anorexia nervosa differs from all others in just how the illness began and in how she deals with it. Tolstoy was right in saying that each individual has his own personal disease, although he did not have the benefit of the scientific advances of the twentieth century. We now can begin to understand how nature and nurture determine the uniqueness of each individual's disease.

The reader who wishes to know more about recent advances in medical genetics and the human genome is directed to *Living with Your Genes* by Hamer and Copeland,[5] Matt Ridley's *Genome, The Autobiography of a Species in 23 Chapters,*[6] and *Principles of Medical Genetics* by Gelehrter, Collins, and Ginsburg.[7]

Environment

People create their own environments to a great extent, and the personalities of individuals tend to determine how others react to them. Children do not merely play a passive role in selecting from and responding to their environment. Their own genetically determined proclivities will have a further effect on their environment.[8]

Once dieting and weight loss have progressed to the point that starvation has set in, it becomes difficult for vulnerable individuals to stop dieting. The response to starvation was studied in conscientious objectors during World War II by Ancel Keys at the University of Minnesota.[9] Profound biological and psychological changes occurred among these people, similar to those observed among patients with anorexia nervosa. The vicious circle that is set in motion is relentless and becomes self-perpetuating. It may be extremely pernicious and lead to chronic anorexia or even death, or the circle may be interrupted and turn to recovery (see Figure 6). There are innate and environmental factors that

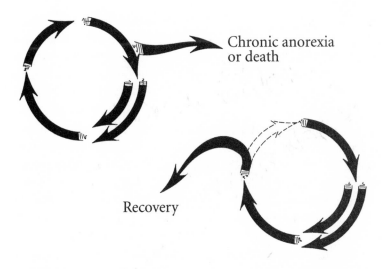

Chronic anorexia
or death

Recovery

Figure 6. Outcomes of anorexia nervosa. From Lucas, AR, Toward the understanding of anorexia nervosa as a disease entity. Mayo Clin Proc, 1981; 56:259.

sustain or ameliorate the disease process. Among the sustaining factors are a severe form of the illness itself, personality factors conducive to maintaining unhealthy eating habits, certain family and interpersonal interactions, the social pressures that value excessive thinness, and inappropriate treatment. On the other hand, a mild form of the illness, effective coping skills, positive family and environmental support, and appropriate treatment may lead to improvement and recovery.

The biopsychosocial model emphasizes that the causative factors interact and synergistically reinforce each other. For each individual they interact in an unique way, but result in a clinical picture that has common features for all those affected. The course of the illness will vary, depending on the sustaining and ameliorating factors described. Outcome may depend very much on the experiences and opportunities in the environment. Some individuals recover spontaneously, or at least without formal treatment. A review of medical records in our community epidemiological study has taught me that it is not unusual for a teenager to lose sufficient weight to qualify for a diagnosis of anorexia nervosa but recover without formal intervention. For these individuals, parents or another influential individual may have provided advice that the teenager was able to accept. At other times, the teenager herself may have realized that what she was doing was irrational and was able to begin eating normally again. Still others may not have had a strong genetic predisposition to develop anorexia nervosa and their natural hunger allowed them to overcome their desire to diet and remain thin. For other individuals, the illness is so severe, and they cling so tenaciously to their distorted ideas that the illness continues, despite the best attempts of family members and professionals to intervene. Some of these become chronic anorexics, doomed to a lifetime of marginal existence, dominated by their chronically starved state. Arthur Crisp, in his book, *Anorexia Nervosa, Let Me Be*,[10] implied that some patients were untreatable and pleaded that they should be allowed to live with their disease in dignity.

Oftentimes the onset of dieting can be unconsciously or consciously motivated by circumstances in the family. The dieting may cease when the precipitating circumstances are resolved, or it may become more extreme when the individual has the biological vulnerability for severe anorexia nervosa. The severity of starvation may trigger that vulnerability, rendering the condition difficult to reverse. Thirteen-year-old Penny's parents had divorced and her father had moved to another city. She and her younger brother remained with their mother. Penny had always been close to her father, but after the divorce he visited infrequently. Penny began to diet and rapidly lost weight. When she went to visit her father during summer vacation he was alarmed by her appearance and sought help for her. Penny's motivation for dieting was to get her father to show her more attention. She also harbored the unrealistic hope that her parents would be reunited. Because her illness was not far advanced it was possible in treatment to deal with her family issues and help her come to a satisfactory conclusion. Penny's hope that her parents would reunite was not realized. Nevertheless, both parents became aware of their daughter's distress, were able to acknowledge her concerns, and arranged for the father to make more frequent visits. Penny no longer had the psychological need to diet and gave up her harmful behavior.

Annette, age 16 years, became preoccupied with counting calories, reading food labels, and avoiding foods containing fats and cholesterol. Although she was still growing, she lost weight and her menstrual periods ceased. The history revealed that her grandfather had recently died of coronary heart disease. His cholesterol level had been elevated and there had been much talk in the family about the consequences of his unhealthy lifestyle. When we discussed her concerns, Annette revealed that she was very worried about her intake of fats and cholesterol in her diet, and she feared that she might develop heart disease like her grandfather. Her serum cholesterol level was measured and was found to be perfectly normal. Her treatment involved working with a dietitian who instructed her in a healthy but sufficient meal plan appropriate for her growth needs and activity during mid-adolescence.

Other girls, and some boys, who have elevated cholesterol levels need careful counseling by a dietician and sometimes by a psychiatrist so they do not inappropriately undernourish themselves during adolescence. Some of these teens may inadvertently develop anorexia nervosa if they are excessively compulsive and fastidious about their diets.

George Hsu hypothesized that dieting, for any reason, provides the entrée to an eating disorder.[11] The more intense the dieting behavior, the greater is the risk of developing an eating disorder. We have already seen that most adolescent girls who start a diet do not develop anorexia nervosa. Hsu further hypothesized that genetic, psychological, biological, personality, and family factors increase the vulnerability to an eating disorder in individuals who diet. He then reviewed the literature pertaining to sociocultural factors, development in adolescence, and identity formation in the female that support the hypothesis. The emphasis on slimness, he says, is intensifying. Even young girls 7 or 8 years of age have concepts about physical attractiveness that are similar to those of adolescents. Girls who are insecure about themselves are most vulnerable to the environmental pressures to diet. Readers who wish to pursue these areas further are directed to Hsu's excellent book.

While the disorder begins most often in young people in whom puberty has begun, it can occur in older individuals as well. Not infrequently it starts in young people beyond high school age, often at the time they are separating from home and family. Our community epidemiologic study has shown that much less commonly it can begin even later in life. When it begins during the adult years, there often is an identifiable precipitant, which may be marriage or the occurrence of an illness. It has manifested in individuals who have had a drinking problem that has led to poor nutrition. In adult life it is frequently associated with a depressive illness. The oldest individual in our community study had onset of the disorder at age 59, an unusually late time for it to begin. This patient did not have a depression and the reason for developing anorexia nervosa was obscure.

Thus, there are many pathways that lead to anorexia nervosa. The illness itself is never fleeting. Once it takes hold it rarely lasts less than six months. More often it continues for several years, either in a mild or severe form. It may last for many years, it may recur at a later time, or it may persist for a lifetime. The outcomes are extremely variable. There are still no ways to predict what the course and outcome will be for a particular individual. My experience has been that most teenagers with the disorder will recover. They tend to miss out on their adolescence, but most make up for their loss and are able to go on with their lives. The follow-up studies that have been done also indicate that most recover, but it often takes a very long time for recovery to occur. These studies are discussed in Chapter 13 on outcome. One must remember that these studies included only patients very severely ill with anorexia nervosa. The less severely ill individuals—those who are seen as outpatients and some of those who may never have come to medical attention—often have a briefer duration of illness.

It is after recovery that the diverse personalities of patients with anorexia nervosa assert themselves again. Just as many roads lead to anorexia nervosa, the roads traveled diverge and go in many directions once the illness is over. Once freed of the constraints of starvation and delayed development, new personality characteristics emerge, and individual skills and capacities become manifest.

Culture

Many cultural forces in our society have a profound effect on girls and young women. Large numbers of young girls are unduly influenced by the ubiquitous media messages to be thin. These influences are pervasive in Western societies and have spread to other developed countries as well. Girls of younger and younger age are constantly influenced by images, models, and performers who are incredulously thin. They emulate these idols by curtailing their nourishment and scrutinizing their own shapes in the mirror. Pre-teens normally have a protuberant abdomen, and this can become an object of abhorrence and disgust to the girl as she matures. The currently popular mode of dress, exposing the abdomen, heightens teens' sensitivity to their figures. Fortunately, most young girls who attempt dieting yield to the biological drive to grow and develop, and they give up their dieting after a short while. Those who persist because of their strong will and determination become anorexic.

The social pressures on women to be thin have been greater than ever in the latter part of the twentieth century, and have not abated. On the contrary, they have become institutionalized in Western culture and have spread to other countries as a result of globalization. The impact of media messages is greatest on girls in their teens. The message glorifying thinness is now widespread. Little wonder that the incidence of anorexia nervosa has steadily been climbing. *Teen Vogue* in the year 2000 is replete with lanky, long-legged models. Their arms and legs are spindly and their abdomens flat. Not one of them sports an average figure. Sara Shandler's book, *Ophelia Speaks*, culled more than 800 writings of adolescent girls from across the country.[12] They wrote personal reflections and poems. The most ubiquitous theme was their body consciousness. More than any other topic, eating disorders appeared in their writing, with 50 of the pieces dealing with their unhealthy relationships with food. One girl has pinups of boys on the walls of her room. But around her mirror she has images of Nadia Anermar, Kate Moss, Amber Valetta, and Shalom Harlow. She wrote, "They are my goals. They are my aspirations. And then I wonder why I hate myself." Shandler describes how girls worry about their anorexic friends, and yet concludes: "In the world of adolescent girls, thinness—sometimes at whatever cost—evokes profound jealousy. We lust for the perfect body. We crave control over our lives. Even when we publicly condemn those who 'control' their food intake, many of us privately admire their 'will power.'"

Some Unusual Cases of Anorexia Nervosa

The case histories we have looked at illustrate the typical onset of anorexia nervosa. In those examples there were the common themes of fear of fatness and the relentless pursuit of thinness. All were girls or young women who strove for perfection but who had impaired self-esteem. Because it occurs most frequently in girls, anorexia nervosa may be overlooked when it occurs in a boy.

Only one in ten anorexics is a boy. Those who develop anorexia nervosa may have a fear of fatness just as girls do. And just as in girls, these boys may begin dieting after their classmates tease them. Some have uniquely false ideas that contribute to their illness. Such was the case of Robert, a 13-year-old eighth grader. At five feet he was somewhat below average in height.

Robert felt inferior to his peers. He was not as skilled as they in athletics, and he tended to be teased by others. Moreover, he was not a good student, though he applied himself to his studies. Some boys teased him about his lack of strength and said that he had weak muscles. He was somewhat chubby, but not obese. Concerned that he had a slight paunch around his waist, he began to feel that his body was flabby and puny. Robert began to exercise and to lift weights. As he exercised more seriously, he began to feel more vigorous and noted that he could run faster. This motivated him to work harder at exercising. Somehow he began to believe that if he weighed less he would become stronger. He consequently restricted what he ate, cutting out fattening foods in particular. He enjoyed some success in losing weight and persisted in the idea that his muscles would become stronger if he ate less and weighed less. Robert kept his thoughts to himself, and did not confide in anyone about his concerns.

At home, there was considerable turmoil in his family. His father was an angry, irritable man who wanted Robert to be athletic, and his mother had once been hospitalized for depression. His siblings were in frequent conflict with their parents.

Robert lost 25 pounds over a six-month period, his weight plummeting to about 100 pounds. He had become progressively weaker, unable to climb stairs without pulling himself up by his arms. His family physician sent him to a pediatric hospital for evaluation. His eyes were puffy and swollen, and his musculature had become wasted. His pulse rate was slow and his potassium level was low. He was suspected of having hypothyroidism or kidney disease. In the hospital he continued to lose weight. After three weeks his weight was only 80 pounds. Because he had become increasingly depressed, he was referred for psychiatric evaluation. When I saw him he described feeling worthless and rotten, and no good to anyone. He was preoccupied about being weak and persisted in the notion that he would get stronger if he exercised and lost more weight. He equated his weakness with flabbiness and fat. He confided that he had been vomiting surreptitiously in the hospital in order to lose more weight.

His medical evaluation, including endocrinological studies, failed to implicate thyroid or kidney disease. Rather, the findings showed the results of starvation. Robert had anorexia nervosa, and he was treated in our psychiatric hospital unit. It was difficult to dissuade Robert from the delusion that becoming thinner would make him stronger. He had to become convinced that nourishing his body was necessary in order to build up his muscles and his strength. As his nutrition improved, his strength and mood improved. Nonetheless, his treatment was a long process fraught with some setbacks before he eventually recovered.

As nutrition improves, thought processes improve as well. As his thinking became more rational Robert became more accepting of our treatment recommendations. His normal appetite returned as well.

The initial trigger had been teasing, compounded by Robert's over-concern about his appearance and competence.

While biological, psychological, and social influences usually work in concert to result in anorexia nervosa, numerous triggers can set off the process of self-starvation. The reason Melissa's dieting began was obscure in her case during the time that she was ill. It was not known until many years later.

Early during my career at Mayo I received a call from a gastroenterologist. He asked me to consult on a young woman of 17 years who had been admitted to the hospital. She was severely starved. When I entered Melissa's room I found her lying in bed. A plastic tube taped to her nose was threaded into her nostril; through it, white liquid nourishment was slowly dripping into her stomach. Her temples and cheeks were sunken. The rims of her orbits were outlined as clearly as on the human skull I had studied in medical school. Her cheek bones protruded prominently beneath her closed, sunken eyes. Her facial skin was tightly drawn over these bones and stretched back from her mouth. She looked like a concentration camp victim. Her pallid complexion gave her a waxy, lifeless appearance. Fragile, bluish, almost transparent limpid lids graced by long, dark lashes covered the prominent globes of her eyes. When she slowly raised them—as if with great effort —her intense dark eyes glistened, asserting that she was still very much alive.

She was by far the most emaciated patient I had ever seen. Her shoulder blades protruded, the vertebrae of her spine and her ribs were clearly visible, and her hip bones stood out prominently. Her stick-like arms and legs were devoid of subcutaneous fat. Her body was more wasted than that of a young woman ravaged by cancer, but her vivid eyes did not show the dull patina of the chronically ill or dying. She turned her doe-like eyes toward me and I noted in them an intensity that bespoke an unextinguished vitality. I introduced myself, and began to ask her some questions. Her answers came in a barely audible whisper.

How the process had started, and what was crucial in her subsequent recovery was obscure at the time. In retrospect, after 30 years, I can see clearly what had happened and what was important in her treatment. Melissa was severely starved, at death's door. Without treatment she surely would soon have died of starvation. Our team of doctors—the internists and psychiatrists—worked feverishly to evaluate what was wrong with Melissa. By providing emergency fluids and electrolytes we kept her alive. But once other medical problems were ruled out and the diagnosis of anorexia nervosa was established, her recovery depended to a large part on her. We provided a safe environment and made life-sustaining food available. We could not have forced her to eat had she refused. It was her will to live and her renewed optimism about the future that led to her recovery.

I am gratified that we did not cause her illness to worsen. Had we forced her to eat more than she was able—had we been in a hurry to give her a diet of 2,000 to 3,000 calories a day and demanded rapid weight gain—she would have balked at being overfed and would have developed a resistance to treatment. Moreover, she might have developed excessive fluid retention that could have pushed her into heart failure. Unfortunately, I have seen this scenario repeated too often at some hospitals to the detriment of anorexic patients.

When she was admitted to the hospital the day before, she had been moribund. Her physicians feared for her life because of her extreme emaciation. Her muscles were wasted, and she barely had the strength to stand. At five feet in height, her weight had dropped below 50 pounds. Indeed, the morning after her hospital admission when she was weighed without her clothes, the scale barely registered at 47½ pounds. Her body temperature was subnormal, her pulse unusually slow, and her blood pressure so low that it was unobtainable with a blood pressure cuff. Her skin was dry and translucent. The only abnormal findings on laboratory examinations, however, were mild anemia, ketosis (a starvation effect involving abnormal buildup of acid ketone bodies in the bloodstream due to breakdown of body fat), and a low potassium level in the blood. All of these could be explained by starvation and occasional vomiting. She had not forced herself to vomit, but her debilitated condition, complicated by the low potassium levels, made her nauseated. Any small amounts of nourishment taken into her empty and shriveled stomach caused irritation and waves of nausea.

Thorough medical evaluations showed no signs of inflammatory bowel disease, no evidence of blood loss, and no tumors or obstruction of the intestinal tract. There was concern that she might have a brain tumor in the area of the pituitary gland or the hypothalamus, which might have interfered with her growth and development and which would have caused vomiting due to pressure on the rest of the brain. Fortunately, none of these ominous concerns were verified, but she began having frequent unexplained loose stools. She continued to feel nauseated and to spit up small amounts of vomitus into an emesis basin by her bed. Consequently, not all of her meager liquid nourishment benefited her. Moreover, we began to suspect that her intestines were not absorbing all of the nourishment provided through the nasogastric tube.

Ultimately the evaluation failed to implicate a medical illness as the cause of her severe undernourishment. It was concluded that she had anorexia nervosa, and we transferred Melissa to our residential treat-

ment unit for adolescents. Her general medical doctors had been startled and worried by her emaciation and had not hesitated to feed her
immediately by stomach tube. They did not want to procrastinate and
risk having her lose even more weight. I believed that tube feeding
should be a last resort. People who have previously been healthy and
who become starved can live for a very long time on their own body
fat. Their metabolism adapts to the reduced caloric intake and becomes
more efficient. Basal metabolism (the rate at which food is burned and
turned into energy by the body) diminishes markedly. This allows the
person to survive on surprisingly little food.

After Melissa was transferred to the psychiatric unit she continued
to have diarrhea, thought to be caused by lactose intolerance. The diarrhea raised new diagnostic questions about an underlying illness, but
this condition may happen when a starved person suddenly is fed supplements containing milk. Moreover, a sudden increase in food can
overwhelm the gastrointestinal tract of a starved person and cause diarrhea. A lactose-free milk product was substituted for the cow's milk
she had been given, and the diarrhea gradually subsided.

After talking with Melissa and finding that she did not fear gaining
weight, I decided to pull out the nasogastric tube. To everyone's surprise, she began to eat everything that was offered, beginning with
small quantities that she could tolerate. This was most unusual for
someone with anorexia nervosa. Moreover, she did not show any of the
distorted eating habits usually associated with the disease. She did not
cut up her food into small pieces or push her food around the plate.
And, remarkably, she did not wipe her buttered toast on a napkin or
surreptitiously drop bits of bread under the table at mealtime. She ate
all the food on her tray, almost greedily, in contrast with the behavior
of other anorexic patients. The other anorexic patients in the unit daw-
dled, sulked, or tried to distract the nurses from their job of supervis-
ing their eating. They were not particularly pleased with the example
that Melissa was setting.

This was not just "honeymoon" behavior or an attempt to eat her
way out of the hospital. As her diarrhea abated and her stomach and
gut readjusted to taking in food, she gradually was able to eat normal
quantities, and her nutritional state improved. Slowly but surely, she
began putting on weight. First, her body became rehydrated; she began

to retain fluids, her skin became turgid, rather than dry and drawn. She was able to become a bit more active; in contrast with the typical anorexic patients, she had not been driven to exercise. Her energy level improved and led to better endurance as her system deposited glycogen in her muscles. Then her face began to fill out a bit, and her bones became less visible as her depleted subcutaneous fat cells began slowly to be restored.

Melissa was an unobtrusive and pleasant patient. Everyone liked her and felt sorry for her because of her waiflike appearance. She was unlike other 17-year-olds. Despite her age she had shown no signs of breast development and had never menstruated. Because of her childlike appearance and demeanor the nurses tended to treat her as much younger than she was. Other patients began to appreciate her as well. Unlike her compatriots on the ward, she caused neither strife nor turmoil.

Melissa was next to the youngest among eight children. Her parents, who farmed in a remote rural area, were older than most. Melissa was a hard worker at home. Unlike her sisters, who preferred to help their mother in the house, she participated in farm chores, often accompanying her father to feed and milk the cows. She was ambitious in school, but lately had become so weak that she could no longer attend. Her father was taciturn. Her mother was more talkative and described family interactions as very pleasant and without strife, noting, "We never have arguments."

Melissa's weight loss and her failure to develop sexually had puzzled her parents. Her mother noted, though, that both she (the mother) and Melissa's oldest sister had been late to develop. None of her siblings were as short as Melissa, however. The most she had ever weighed was 86 pounds, two years earlier, but then she had looked well nourished. She had almost suddenly lost about 20 pounds. Medical evaluation by her local physician did not reveal a cause. Subsequently, she was twice hospitalized at the distant university hospital. The first evaluation provided no better answers. The second time the diagnosis of anorexia nervosa was suspected when Melissa was admitted to the psychiatric unit there. Questions by a psychiatrist about sexual issues made her uncomfortable and she asked her parents to take her home. As she continued to lose weight, her parents took her to a new doctor in town who urgently referred her to Mayo.

Melissa's weight recovery in our hospital was unremarkable. She ate what was served to her without protest and gained weight steadily. As her nourishment improved, so did her general health, confirming that she had no underlying physical illness. Her level of energy increased remarkably, and she participated in activities without overdoing them. In every way she behaved like a preadolescent. Her physical appearance, underdeveloped as she was, made her seem more like a 12-year-old than 17.

She eventually was able to choose her own meals without difficulty, and in due time, when her normal but immature body was fully restored, it was felt that she could return home. In those days, we were able to treat patients in the hospital for months, assuring their recovery. She returned to the care of her hometown physician in her small farming community. Periodic follow-up by him confirmed that she continued to do well.

Thirteen years later I located Melissa and contacted her by telephone to learn how she was doing. She was working at that time as a nurse's aide in a small community not far from her parents' farm. She told me that she was able to maintain her increased weight and had finished high school after she left the hospital. I asked if she ever developed and matured physically. She said, "Oh, yes, I got my periods when I was 22, and now I'm a living doll! I have a boyfriend, too." I was curious to know what, if anything, she remembered about the time she was in the hospital. She said it had been a frightening time for her. She had felt miserable for some time before, but she had recovered and was now a happy young woman. I explained that I wanted to learn more about the causes of anorexia nervosa and that in her case, we had no idea what led to her becoming so undernourished. It seemed evident that when she was in the hospital she wanted to get well again. Did she remember anything that might help us understand why she began losing weight? She said, "Oh, yes, my brother was sexually abusing me, and I wanted him to leave me alone. But I didn't dare tell my parents, and I wouldn't tell anybody about it in the hospital when I was 17." She had stopped eating to keep him away.

Some claim that most, if not all, girls and women who develop an eating disorder have been sexually abused. The fact is that sexual abuse is common in our society. We used to think it happened only in Appalachia or in backward uneducated communities. In reality, it occurs everywhere, even in seemingly exemplary families. Definitions of sexual abuse vary widely. There is a broad spectrum of behavior, ranging from normal sexual exploration among children to forced activity by a much older person. Where does one draw the line in defining sexual abuse? Children in school these days are taught about "good touch" and "bad touch." The distinction can be difficult to make.

Epidemiological studies of women vary greatly in the prevalence rates of sexual abuse they experienced as children. The rates varied from 6 percent to 62 percent in 19 different U.S. and Canadian samples studied, with the average rate being 23 percent, or 1 in 5 women. Among 13 studies in men, the rates range from 3 percent to 30 percent, with an average rate of 10 percent, or 1 in 10.[13] On the whole, sexual abuse is underreported. The discrepant rates may be accounted for by different definitions of sexual abuse, by real differences among various segments of the population or in different cultural groups, and by variations in the methodology of the studies.

A study comparing the rates of childhood sexual abuse in women with anorexia nervosa, borderline personality disorder, or no psychiatric disorder found that the women with borderline personality disorder had suffered repeated sexual abuse whereas the anorexic and normal groups had experienced rare events of sexual abuse.[14] It is likely that women with anorexia nervosa have experienced sexual abuse no more frequently than other women in the general population. Women with bulimic disorders are more likely to have been abused than women with anorexia nervosa.

Melissa's story illustrates that things are not always what they seem to be. When she was first admitted to the hospital she was extremely emaciated. It seemed inconceivable that in modern times anyone could go as long as she did without receiving necessary medical help. Because her body was far more severely starved than any of the anorexic patients we had seen during the preceding years, it was reasonable to look for other causes. Other diseases were eliminated by the medical evaluations. She was not depressed. Moreover, appetite loss and weight loss from depression do not progress that far. Melissa had an atypical form of anorexia nervosa without the psychological features that usually accompany it. She did not express a fear of becoming fat, and seemed to recognize that she was abnormally thin. Much to everyone's surprise, Melissa behaved differently from other anorexic patients who vehemently resist eating the food they are offered. She was willing, even eager, to eat.

Had Melissa been in a program with a rigid protocol for the treatment of anorexia nervosa, her stomach tube might have remained in place. That she was willing and able to eat regular food would not have been apparent so quickly. Additionally, she would have been started on progressively larger meals after she had gained a certain amount of weight on liquid feedings. Had she not gained a required amount of weight each day, her freedom and activities would have been restricted. As it was, in our program, she gained weight over time but certainly not every day. Some days she would gain a bit, but on another day she might lose a half-pound. Had we punished or restricted her for this natural day-by-day weight fluctuation, she would justifiably have become angry or oppositional, and effective treatment would have been compromised. Thus, the illness can be reinforced by inappropriate treatment. Setting unrealistic expectations would have discouraged and antagonized her, complicating a process that she was well able to carry out at her own pace. In retrospect, it was evident that Melissa felt free to eat again, and she was no longer trying to prevent her sexuality and womanhood from emerging. At the time of her illness she was quite unable to express such thoughts, and the sexual advances her brother had made were a deep, dark secret she would not confide even to her mother or her closest friend. When Melissa returned home, her brother had already moved away and she no longer had to fear him. Also, she was more mature and confident in herself and could successfully ward off any unwelcome advances.

The reason for Melissa's small stature and her total lack of sexual development by age 17 were not fully understood at the time she was in the hospital. The information obtained many years later showed that Melissa had continued to grow and gain for a number of years. There had been a delay in her growth and sexual maturation. She did experience puberty and adolescence, just years later than usual. Fortunately, the growth plates in her long bones had not yet closed, and she continued to grow in stature. When a young child fails to gain weight, growth is often stunted. It has been shown clearly that catch-up growth will occur if weight is restored before the ends of the bones are fused. Roxane Pfeiffer and I, studying the records of 71 patients with anorexia nervosa, found that when weight loss occurs after the process of puberty had started, growth in height will not be stunted.[15] Melissa, as her outcome was to prove, had delayed growth during her pre-pubertal time of weight loss, but was able to grow a full three inches after the age of 18.

Melissa's story illustrates how individual patients' histories differ one from another. Sometimes a life event or series of events can lead to the disorder; at other times no such precipitating event is found. Without doubt, some people are highly vulnerable to the disease, and little is required to precipitate it. Most girls will never develop the disease, no matter how compelling their stress. The differences among the patients with many different forms of anorexia nervosa should dictate individualization in their treatment. In Melissa's case, her severe malnutrition had first to be addressed because she was close to death from starvation. Once her precarious physical state was corrected, she could be given general guidelines about her nutritional requirements. More important, her natural hunger took over once she was in a safe environment, and she could begin eating again with little supervision. Her sexual abuse was not addressed because it was not known. She was effectively able to cope with it herself once she had recovered from her illness. Moreover, her brother, the source of the sexual abuse, was no longer at home when she returned.

CHAPTER FIVE

The Signs of Trouble

In this chapter I describe some of the behaviors and physical signs that occur early in the onset of anorexia nervosa. Included is a checklist for parents that provides guidance about evaluating which symptoms and signs may be observed for a time and which warrant prompt action.

Parents of adolescents are often confronted by behaviors that are difficult to understand. They may be unable to distinguish those that are to be expected from those that signal trouble. This is particularly true when a daughter is showing symptoms that may denote an eating disorder. Her parents are torn between hoping that the behavior is a transient phase and fearing that it represents something serious. Friends or relatives may give well-meaning but conflicting advice about what to do. This was the dilemma confronting Frances's mother.

Frances was a young woman who inadvertently developed anorexia nervosa as a result of her participation in athletics. Living in rural Wisconsin, a senior in high school, Frances took up running and began to treat this sport as seriously as she did her studies. As she achieved some success in her running, she worked increasingly hard by training more and more. She was good at it, and she wanted to become the best.

I received a call from her distraught mother who explained that Frances had been losing weight but always managed to avoid the topic whenever her mother brought it up. While Frances seemed to have gotten thin during the summer months, her mother reported that Frances's sports physical exam at the beginning of the school year was satisfactory. Frances continued to be a strong runner, but her weight loss continued, so the mother took her to her family physician after the fall semester. He indicated that he couldn't find anything wrong and attributed her loss of menstrual periods to running. Still worried about Frances's weight loss and social withdrawal, the mother sought out a psychologist, who said that Frances had an eating disorder. Frances was unwilling to acknowledge that there was a problem and refused to see the psychologist again. She supported her conviction by pointing out that she was eating three meals a day and didn't want to harm her body. Never one to express her feelings freely, she had become more isolated and irritable, seeming to shut her mother out of her life.

Frances was indeed functioning well in other respects—she had excellent academic grades and enjoyed a small circle of friends. Her mother felt frustrated and asked me what to do to get help for Frances. A friend had suggested a stay in a hospital in a nearby city that had an eating disorder program, but she was certain that Frances would refuse. I told her that Frances's symptoms indicated that she needed to be seen for an evaluation and that I would be glad to see her. Her mother first needed to have a serious talk with her daughter, to tell her frankly how concerned she was about her, and she needed to tell her that she had called me for an appointment. She should also tell her that I would be frank with her, I would want to know her own view of the situation, and I would make recommendations that she could consider. I advised Frances's mother that hospitalization is not the first option in treatment, certainly not before the patient has a thorough evaluation. We would need to determine how large the problem was and whether Frances simply needed some advice or active treatment. I assured her mother that I would discuss my impressions with Frances and make recommendations that she could accept or not.

The appointment was arranged for Frances. She was soft-spoken and brief in her responses, showing little emotion. Of average height, at 5 feet 6 inches, she confided that she had weighed 122 pounds at age 15, before she lost about 20 pounds. She had eliminated red meats from her diet and reduced her fat intake. She was exercising regularly at the "Y," running on a treadmill, bicycling, and using a stair-climber. While not emaciated, she showed physical signs of moderate starvation. She acknowledged that she felt cold much of the time and was frequently fatigued. Her scalp hair had been falling out when she brushed it. She volunteered no additional information but listened with heightened interest when I discussed the process of adolescent growth, and described the physiological effects of starvation.

I had her see the dietitian with whom I worked, who determined that her daily intake amounted to no more than 1,000 calories. Although consuming three meals a day, Frances was using only fat-free foods, and she had eliminated all visible fat from her meals. She ate limited amounts of chicken and fish, consuming chiefly vegetables and fruits. As a start, the dietitian prescribed a meal plan consisting of a greater variety of foods, and amounting to 1,300 calories daily, allowing her some food choices based on her likes and dislikes. Frances agreed to return to see us, and we saw her every two weeks throughout the spring and summer to work on improving her eating habits. While she remained aloof and distant toward me, she made an effort to follow the recommendations and faithfully kept a food diary. Her daily records documented a gradual increase in amounts, as advised by the dietitian, and a broadening of her food choices. She was more comfortable discussing things with the dietitian than with me, often asking her meaningful questions about the nutritional composition and caloric content of various foods. She lost no more weight, and then was able to begin gaining weight steadily.

Her psychotherapy at first involved educational explanations of the physical effects of weight gain. Frances needed much reassurance that the associated abdominal discomfort with feelings of bloating was expected and not harmful. She was able to express the anxiety that she felt about this process to the dietitian and to me. As she became more confident and less afraid to eat, discussions focused more on her school activities and particularly on her plans for college. Her parents understandably were concerned about whether Frances would be able to maintain her physical improvement and normalized eating habits at college. She would be away from home and would be without her frequent therapy sessions. Frances had several options for college, including a large university some distance from her home, and a small college nearby. Her best friend planned to go to the university, but Frances eventually decided on the small college. The dietitian reviewed the practical aspects of eating meals at the school, including what foods

Frances could keep in the small refrigerator in her dormitory room and what she could eat at the college cafeteria. Frances was eating comfortably enough to make us feel that she could manage this.

The question arose of whether she should see someone at the school for counseling. After discussing the possibilities, Frances decided that she would prefer to return to see us during Thanksgiving vacation in November and until then to keep in touch by mail, or by telephone, if necessary. It might seem that arranging for therapy at college would have been the most supportive thing to do. However, once a person has developed a trusting relationship with a therapist, it is difficult to shift that allegiance to someone new. Frances felt confident enough to cope with a new situation at school, but preferred to be able to call on us to maintain contact on an infrequent basis. This avoided the necessity of having her review her story all over again with another person and of developing a relationship with someone new. She had become familiar with our approach and treatment philosophy and didn't need a new orientation. As it turned out, Frances was able to manage her eating well enough that she lost only a few pounds after beginning college. She came to see us at Thanksgiving and reported that she found her schoolwork challenging and requiring considerable effort. Her relationship with her roommate had turned out to be disastrous because the roommate's habits were radically different from her own. This resulted in frequent tearful calls to her mother and reactivated feelings of self-doubt and insecurity that she had not revealed before. Many nonanorexic freshman college students who have led sheltered lives experience similar culture shock when they first go away to school. She persisted through this difficult time, however, and was able to weather the rest of her freshman year.

By the following autumn, when Frances began her second year at college, her weight had reached 130 pounds. She had befriended three compatible students, and they decided to room together in a dormitory "quad." She developed some symptoms of depression, not unusual for someone who is recovering from anorexia nervosa. After discussing her feelings with me she agreed to take an antidepressant medication for a period of time. The depression gradually lifted as her junior year in college brought increasing success for her academically and socially.

Frances, at last, had made a recovery.

The signs of trouble that signal the onset of anorexia nervosa fall into two categories: behavioral and physical.

Changes in Behavior

The most obvious behavioral change involves eating behavior and attitude toward food. Eating smaller quantities and eliminating foods thought to be fattening are the most common manifestations of this change. The girl developing anorexia nervosa may refuse second helpings and avoid foods that contain fat. She may begin to cut her food up into small pieces and eat more slowly. Quite commonly she leaves some food on her plate or discards it clandestinely. She may avoid coming to the table when the family eats together. Since it is common for family members to eat separately or on the run, parents may not notice changes in a child's eating behavior at first. The child may skip breakfast or not eat lunch at school. Often she will eliminate foods containing sugar, avoiding sweets and desserts. Sometimes, however, she may substitute candy for a regular meal to suppress her hunger and to provide a quick source of energy. She may use quantities of mustard or other condiments to flavor small amounts of bland food. Often, an anorexic girl will chew gum as a substitute for eating. Changes in eating patterns to vegetarianism are not unusual. She may rationalize that this is for health reasons or because she doesn't want to eat animals, when the real reason is to eliminate fat and to reduce calories. During puberty it may be difficult to distinguish developmentally normal behavioral changes from pathological behavior. It is the severity and persistence of the behavior that suggest anorexia nervosa.

Sometimes such changes in eating behavior may be readily apparent, but more often the girl who is developing anorexia nervosa becomes secretive about her eating behavior. She may make a show of participating in one family meal a day when she eats heartily, but she will avoid her other meals. Not infrequently, when asked about how she has eaten, she will describe one perfectly adequate meal but fail to mention that she starved herself for several days before.

It is common for the emerging anorexic to show remarkable interest in food, cooking, and nutrition. This may include reading culinary magazines and cookbooks, collecting recipes, and memorizing the caloric content of foods. She may take an interest in cooking and baking for her family and in encouraging others to eat.

The second behavioral change involves increased activity and exercise. Usually the girl who is developing anorexia nervosa begins to invest more energy in all her activities. She begins to walk faster, to participate in more activities, and to complete them more quickly. These behaviors may become frenetic. She may eagerly do housework and other tasks that she avoided before. She may get up early in the morning in order to do these tasks or to do schoolwork. Her activity usually involves planned physical exercise. This may take the form of increased involvement in sports or engaging in an exercise program involving calisthenics. Usually she will set increasingly higher goals for herself, doing more and more sit-ups or jumping jacks each day. She may avoid sitting down and spend much of her time standing. She may be restless when she is required to sit still, and she may engage in isometric exercises.

While many anorexics—particularly true in the past—only restrict their food intake, some also vomit to lose weight. They may use diet pills, laxatives, or diuretics to accomplish greater weight loss. Some eat intermittently when overcome by hunger cravings, and even overeat; then they vomit or purge with laxatives or enemas to rid themselves of the food they have eaten. These behaviors are done secretly and may go unnoticed by family members unless they are alert to the possibility.

Other behavioral changes include social withdrawal from friends and family. The girl developing anorexia nervosa may begin spending more time alone, isolating herself in her room. Such behavior is common among most children during the early teens when they begin to turn away from their parents, wanting their privacy, and asserting their independence. The typical early teenage girl turns to her friends whereas the one developing anorexia nervosa distances herself from her peers as well as from her parents. Girls who are depressed similarly show withdrawn and isolative behavior, but they lose interest in their surroundings and in their schoolwork as well. They slow down physically. In contrast, the anorexic girl is active physically and may spend hours doing her schoolwork conscientiously when she is alone in her room. She would like to have friends, but she feels threatened by her age-mates' behavior. She feels uncomfortable about their seeking independence and their experimenting with risky behaviors. Many of her peers are trying out alcohol and drugs and beginning to engage in sexual activity. She disapproves of these behaviors and may be frightened of them.

Her thoughts and feelings are changing as well. Many are unexpressed to others and remain private thoughts. In fact, she becomes more reluctant to share many of her concerns with others, particularly with her parents. Some of her thoughts she expresses freely, however. These have to do with her image of herself. She says things like, "I'm fat!" or "I'm so ugly!" She insists that "All my friends are thinner than I am." Such comments provide clues to her preoccupation with her body image. Perhaps a majority of teenage girls voice such concerns. By themselves, they need not cause alarm, but when they are acted on by excessive dieting they signal overconcern about appearance.

None of these changes alone indicates the likelihood of anorexia nervosa. Some of these behaviors occur in one person and not in another. It is the presence of several, leading to the physical changes, that signal the disorder.

Physical Changes

Among the physical changes, weight loss is of course the first and most enduring sign of trouble. The younger the child, the less likely there is to be actual weight loss at first. Children who develop anorexia nervosa before puberty or early in the pubertal stages of development tend not to lose weight rapidly, but they fail to continue gaining weight at the expected rate. Their growth in stature slows along with this failure to gain weight. This trend is seen in boys as well as in girls. Once they are well into puberty, actual weight loss may be slow or rapid. The speed with which it occurs depends on the previous nutritional state and the severity of food restriction. Most often the change is at first subtle and may go unnoticed from week to week or even from month to month. Once dieting has become established and food intake is further curtailed, weight comes off more rapidly. Among girls who have started menstruating and are well along into puberty, the process usually takes some months. Less often the decline is precipitous and readily apparent, when eating is drastically restricted.

Along with the weight loss, inadequate nourishment causes body processes to change: heart rate slows and blood pressure drops. What little food the person eats is retained in the stomach longer as the churning activity of digestion slows down. This may result in the feeling of fullness, bloating, and stomachache. Food is digested more slowly and thoroughly in the bowels, resulting in constipation. Bowel movements become small and infrequent.

Undernourishment leads to fatigue. Anorexic girls resist this and overcome their fatigue by pushing themselves to remain active. Their ability to concentrate becomes impaired and they may be unable to do their schoolwork efficiently. They often complain of headache, a sign that blood sugar levels may be low. Their skin becomes dry and their hair becomes brittle and thin. When they brush their scalp hair, it may come out in bunches. The palms of their hands may take on an orange hue, signaling an abnormal buildup of carotene.

Among premenarchal girls the onset of menstruation is delayed as long as they remain significantly underweight. Among girls who have begun to menstruate, weight loss leads to cessation of periods, usually after a critical amount of weight has been lost. Less often menses may cease before much weight is lost. Breast development and growth of pubic hair may be delayed. In boys there is an analogous delay in pubertal development.

The following checklist provides some of the prominent changes that may appear at the onset of anorexia nervosa. The physiological changes that accompany chronic undernutrition and starvation are discussed in greater depth in Chapter 9.

CHECKLIST FOR PARENTS
Food avoidance
Marked change in food preference
Avoidance of family meals
Excessive interest in food, cooking, and recipes
Excessive physical activity and exercise
Unexplained disappearance of food
Secretive vomiting
Use of diet pills, laxatives, or diuretics
Social withdrawal
Failure to gain weight during the growth years

Unexplained weight loss
Delay in onset of menstrual periods
Cessation of periods after they have begun

One or more of these behavioral symptoms and physical signs may signal the onset of an eating disorder. If the changes are mild they warrant watching. However, if they are severe and lasting, they should be taken seriously and the child should have a prompt evaluation.

The abuse of medication calls for immediate attention.

Social withdrawal, when associated with other symptoms, may indicate an eating disorder, but it is more likely a symptom of depression.

Failure to gain weight during the preadolescent or adolescent years can be watched for a few months, but if it persists or if there is actual weight loss, an evaluation is indicated. If weight loss is mild and of brief duration and unaccompanied by behavioral symptoms, it may be watched for a few weeks, even for a month or two. But if it persists or is accompanied by other symptoms, an evaluation should be sought quickly.

Commonly, some time is required before periods are established regularly so loss of periods during adolescence is usually benign. When associated with weight loss, however, it should be investigated medically.

When confronted with some of these signs parents should talk with their teens. Maintaining good communications and being available when one's child is willing to talk is a key to good parenting. Parents can err on the side of ignoring serious symptoms, hoping that they will pass, or overreact and nag their child about eating. When, for example, vomiting or the use of laxatives is suspected, the teen should be confronted directly. It is important for parents to tell their teens frankly that they are concerned about harmful behaviors and that they expect them to stop. Sometimes these behaviors can be nipped in the bud before they become ingrained. If the teen is unwilling or unable to stop inappropriate dieting or other harmful behavior, professional help is necessary. Parents should not be afraid to ask their daughter how much she weighs. Secrecy can lead to deception that becomes habitual. On the other hand, it is not helpful for parents to react punitively or with anger. When that happens parents need professional guidance to help them deal with their feelings.

CHAPTER SIX

What to Expect in an Evaluation

Parents of a teenager whose behavior suggests anorexia nervosa are faced with a dilemma. Should they be patient and hope that the problem will resolve itself, or should they confront their child and insist on getting prompt professional help? As with other aspects of child rearing, there is no easy answer because children differ one from another. The ways in which eating disorders begin are quite variable. Whether changes in eating habits will persist is impossible to predict at the start. Knowing one's child and being able to talk freely with her are the best ways of assuring that a parent remains in touch with what is going on. When a pre-teen or early teenager balks at certain foods or seems to become finicky in her eating habits, it is usually judicious to wait a while before reacting. Most often such behaviors are transient. When the behaviors persist, however, and it becomes apparent that she is continuing to curtail the amount of food she is eating to the point that she is losing weight, it is time to have a talk with her. This is particularly indicated when the behavior is coupled with a notable change in demeanor. The parent should ask why the child is avoiding food and express concern, without alarm, that this eating change is unhealthy. The parents should explain that it can interfere with normal growth during adolescence, provide too little energy for physical activities, and interfere with efficient thinking and concentration. Some children will respond to reason at this early stage of dieting and be willing to stop their harmful behavior.

Quite likely a parent will receive a negative response to such questions with the child unwilling to talk about it, or saying, "I'm not hungry" or "What I eat is my own business." A parent should persist by bringing the subject up another time but not allowing the discussion to escalate into an argument. Parents should not be misled into providing special foods or diet foods for their daughter but should expect her to eat what everyone else in the family eats.

Sally, a 14-year-old ballet dancer, began dieting and lost some weight. Her mother had a good relationship with her and had a talk with Sally about her dieting. She pointed out that she needed energy to perform, and she needed to nourish her body to remain healthy and to continue to grow. She set a realistic weight below which Sally would not be allowed to continue her ballet lessons. Sally understood, and met these expectations, even though she would have liked nothing better than to lose more weight. She trusted her mother enough to know that her advice was good. Although she disagreed with her, she did not want to lose her opportunity to continue ballet.

Not everyone is as responsible as Sally or as accepting of parental advice. When it becomes evident that a daughter is failing to gain weight over a period of months or is even losing weight, the situation needs closer attention. If she has become evasive and secretive about her weight and eating habits, a competent evaluation is needed.

Whom to Turn To and What Steps to Take

The first person to turn to is one's family physician or pediatrician. A medical evaluation is essential because there can be many reasons for weight loss. The medical history, a physical examination, and perhaps some simple laboratory tests will generally show if there are causes for the weight loss other than anorexia nervosa. These causes include depression, hyperthyroidism, diabetes, and inflammatory bowel disease, among others. A careful history of how the girl's eating habits have changed and how much weight she has lost will be obtained. The medical history, or the story of how the disorder evolved, is by far the most important element in making the diagnosis. A thorough physical examination is a necessary part of evaluating any patient who may have anorexia nervosa. Signs of weight loss with loss of body fat and perhaps wasting of the musculature are the most evident features. Extensive laboratory tests are usually unnecessary to establish the correct diagnosis. Resting energy expenditure, or the basal metabolic rate, is sometimes measured and may help to confirm the diagnosis. It is invariably low in undernourished anorexic patients. It will also provide accurate information about the patient's caloric needs.

Psychological testing does not help to make the diagnosis of anorexia nervosa. Used selectively, it may provide clues to planning treatment strategies by documenting the patient's intelligence and personality characteristics. It may confirm that an individual is overachieving or working at her capacity in school. In a practical sense, however, the information gained directly in talking with the patient is of most use in guiding how treatment should proceed.

It is most helpful if parents can bring a record of their daughter's prior heights and weights, which can be plotted on a growth chart. The chart graphically depicts physical growth over time, and accurate measurements of height and weight can set a baseline for future comparison. The growth chart is a valuable aid in documenting the growth pattern of a child. Height and weight are plotted on separate curves, based on standards for the U.S. population. Percentiles are indicated to show the norms and variability among children. There are separate growth charts for girls and for boys. Most children continue to grow in height within about the same percentile whether they are tall, average, or short. Girls tend to slow their growth and stop growing in stature soon after age 15; boys generally continue to grow until age 18 or later. Weight also progresses in a somewhat predictable manner, although not as consistently as height. Overweight children tend to remain so, and thin children are likely to remain thin. When there is a notable change in the weight percentile over time there may be a medical reason, or a child's eating habits may have changed markedly. Although girls stop growing taller around the age of 15, their weight normally continues to increase until age 18 as their bodies develop sexually.

Most pediatricians and family physicians are competent to make the diagnosis of anorexia nervosa. They often treat patients in the early stages of the illness when the process can often be reversed. Treatment may include seeing a dietitian. Sometimes the patient is referred to a child and adolescent psychiatrist or to another professional experienced with eating disorders. This is recommended when the patient resists treatment or when there are apparent conflicts in the family. Regardless of which professional provides the treatment, working with an anorexic patient takes much time. Parents should ask what experience the physician has had in evaluating and treating patients with eating disorders. The distribution of experienced professionals varies from community to community. Finding one can be challenging. Ask your physician for a recommendation. If there are no experienced professionals available in the community, it may be necessary to go to a university medical center or a large medical clinic. The most comprehensive listing of experienced professionals for this disorder is the membership directory of the Academy for Eating Disorders.[1] Members of that organization must have certain academic, training, and clinical credentials. The organization includes members from several disciplines, including psychiatry, psychology, dietetics, and social work. Of course, meeting the required criteria does not assure competence, but membership in the Academy is of help in finding an experienced professional. A personal recommendation is also useful. Ultimately, parents' own impressions of the individual are important if they are to have confidence and trust in this person.

What kind of professionals are qualified to diagnose and treat patients with anorexia nervosa? First, a physician with a medical degree (M.D. or D.O.) must do the evaluation. A psychiatrist is most likely to be the medical specialist most qualified to treat eating disordered patients. The psychiatrist may carry out the treatment alone or in cooperation with an internist or pediatrician depending on the age of the patient. In my practice I carried out much of the evaluation and treatment myself, sometimes in consultation with a pediatrician or internist (endocrinologist or gastroenterologist) depending on the patient's symptoms. I found it valuable to work with a very experienced dietitian who guided the nutritional aspects of the treatment. The psychiatrist or other physician may provide much of the direct treatment to the patient—that is, general guidance, psychotherapy, and medication—or another therapist may provide the psychotherapy. This may be a clinical psychologist with a Ph.D. degree or a psychiatric social worker. Psychologists holding a master's degree may also have been trained to treat patients with eating disorders and may be effectively involved as long as they are supervised by a Ph.D. level psychologist or a physician. There are other therapists such as nurse specialists who have gained experience in treating patients with eating disorders. In selecting someone to treat your daughter or other family member, it is reasonable to ask about the potential therapist's credentials and experience in treating eating disorders. The recommendations of other professionals in your community who know the work of the therapist in question are invaluable. The involvement of a knowledgeable physician is necessary because of the many possible physical aspects of the disease.

In most instances, when first seeing an adolescent for evaluation, I found it best to meet with the parents and patient together to get a sense of what their concerns are and how they interact. Frequently these concerns had not been expressed clearly at home. Airing these concerns helps the patient to understand what the parents are worried about and gives the patient a chance to state her views. I then would see them separately to glean more detailed information.

With pre-pubertal children who are balking at eating or showing other deviations in their eating patterns, the parents should be counseled to avoid making an issue of what and how much the children should eat. They should make a variety of foods available. Frequently young children will favor certain foods and avoid others for periods of time. They may refuse food as a means of opposing their parents. Most often these behaviors do not last long. Most children will soon give in to their hunger, particularly when they see that their parents are not distressed over their food refusal.

With adolescents the problem often has become more fixed, as they are determined to lose weight to attain the slim image they desire. The challenge in beginning to work with adolescents is twofold: to help the parents to cope more effectively with the situation, and to convince the adolescent that there is a problem she needs to deal with. The adolescent will often complain that her parents are pressuring her too much to eat. Doing this will not help. On the contrary, it will make her even more determined to have her own way. The interaction between the adolescent and her parents has usually become highly charged emotionally. It is frightening to see one's daughter starving herself. Nonetheless, parents should be advised to back off and to avoid fighting about the food issues. They should not attempt to force her to eat since that usually makes matters worse. Instead, they should let their daughter know that they are very concerned, but leave the food issues in the hands of the professional treating her. That person is not emotionally involved and can more effectively set expectations.

We look at specific aims and principles of treatment in Chapter 12. In this chapter we start at the beginning of the treatment—with the evaluation. The evaluation sets the stage and blends imperceptibly into treatment. Specific treatment strategies then follow from the evaluation.

Parents of a child or adolescent who is showing signs of developing an eating disorder are faced with a mixture of emotions. They are likely to be concerned, to feel guilty, and to feel angry. A parent's natural instinct when her daughter is restricting her food intake is to be worried and to want to feed her. Parents often wonder why it has happened and ask themselves, "What did I do to cause this?" They may wonder if an eating problem in their family or their spouse's family was inherited. All of these thoughts may give rise to guilt and self-recrimination. When a daughter fails to heed a parent's attempts to nurture—and particularly when she engages in injurious behavior, such as self-induced vomiting—feelings of disbelief and anger are likely to be aroused. The daughter who has the eating problem likewise harbors mixed feelings. Foremost, she wants to be left alone, and she resents parental admonitions or encouragement to eat more. She may also feel guilty about causing her parents grief and expense, but these feelings often do not become manifest until long after the onset of the problem.

It is the task of the professional evaluating the situation to help sort out these feelings and to relieve inappropriate guilt and anger. In the past parents were often blamed for being overcontrolling and for making all decisions for the child who becomes anorexic. The child would be compliant and conforming. Eventually she would rebel by controlling her eating, that aspect of her life that her parents could not control. While this was an interesting hypothesis of causation, most families in which anorexia nervosa occurs do not fit that pattern. Many different styles of parenting have been observed. Parents do not cause the problem. The causes are many and complex, as we saw in Chapter 4. Recriminations and blame are not helpful. Rather, a plan should be made to deal effectively with the disorder.

Summary

1. When should we seek an evaluation?

   When weight loss is inappropriate for age and developmental level or when harmful behaviors persist.

2. What is involved in an evaluation?

   History taking from the parents and from the patient to get a chronological story of physical and behavioral changes. This includes an exploration of the patient's attitude toward her weight loss, her view of her body, and her motivation for treatment. We look for what might have triggered it, what she is struggling with, and with whom she is having conflicts.

   A medical evaluation is essential to eliminate other causes of weight loss and to determine physical complications.

   Some laboratory tests may be indicated; this depends on the severity and stage of the illness.

   Other medical specialists may be involved in the evaluation if there are special medical concerns.

3. Whom will we see for an evaluation?

   A physician—pediatrician, family practitioner, or internist—does the initial evaluation. That person may request consultation by an endocrinologist, gastroenterologist, or psychiatrist.

4. What comes after the evaluation?

   The physician, with the parents and patient, develops a treatment plan. Once the treatment plan is implemented the physician may provide follow-up or turn the direct treatment over to a psychiatrist, psychologist or other experienced therapist.

5. What if the parents need guidance?

   The parents may be involved in counseling by a psychiatrist, psychologist, or social worker.

These guidelines provide a very general framework for understanding the evaluation. Note that both the evaluation and treatment should be highly individualized and that no rigid plan will fit all.

CHAPTER SEVEN

Making the Diagnosis

Serious efforts to set specific criteria for diagnosing psychiatric illnesses began in the 1960s, particularly at Washington University in St. Louis. To make the study of psychiatric disorders more objective, research diagnostic criteria were proposed so that researchers could study patients who shared the same characteristics.[1] These criteria eventually evolved into standards promulgated by the American Psychiatric Association (APA). The APA criteria have become the accepted standard and are now used worldwide. Periodically they are modified and updated to reflect research advances. These criteria are published in the fourth edition of the *Diagnostic and Statistical Manual of Mental Disorders* (*DSM-IV*). The diagnostic criteria for anorexia nervosa include (1) refusal to maintain body weight at a minimally normal body weight for age and height (weight loss to 85% of expected weight); (2) intense fear of gaining weight or becoming fat, even though underweight; (3) disturbance in the way in which one's body weight or shape is experienced; and (4) amenorrhea in women (loss of three or more consecutive menstrual periods).[2]

Some patients with anorexia nervosa only restrict their food intake and exercise to lose weight. Others may also vomit or purge (use laxatives, diuretics, or enemas) to accomplish weight loss. Some have eating binges periodically when they eat a large quantity of food and then vomit or purge to rid themselves of unwanted food.

The *DSM-IV* characteristics sound much more scientific than say-

ing "A previously healthy person who has lost a great deal of weight because of not eating enough." Yet that is really what the diagnosis of
anorexia nervosa comes down to. There is the additional implication
that the person who lost weight does not have a realistic sense of what
her body looks like and that she does not want to resume normal eating because of her fear of becoming fat. These factors play a role in the
motivation to diet.

Diagnosis in medicine has two chief purposes. The first is to charac-
terize an illness with a particular group of symptoms that have a common cause. The second is to allow for treating the condition in a rational way so as to achieve a predictable outcome. Strep throat is
manifested by fever, a deeply red inflammation of the throat, and severe
sore throat. The diagnosis is confirmed by culturing the bacterium,
Streptococcus, Group A. The illness is effectively treated with penicillin.
This is the neat scheme that physicians like to work with. Unfortunately,
many illnesses, psychiatric disorders, and particularly anorexia nervosa,
do not behave in so neat and predictable a fashion. There are many reasons—some well understood, and others not so well understood—for a
person to begin dieting inappropriately. The many factors that lead to
this inappropriate dieting have been discussed in Chapter 4. Case histories illustrate different ways in which the process starts.

In the United Kingdom the diagnostic criteria are expressed somewhat differently: (1) significant weight loss; (2) an endocrine disorder
as manifested by amenorrhea in women; (3) a psychological disturbance manifested by an irrational fear of fatness.[3] The words and concepts are somewhat different, but they describe the same patients. So, it
can be seen that the criteria are all somewhat arbitrary. Indeed, com-
mittees have changed them every few years—not so much because the
patients have changed but because evolving knowledge has allowed us
to refine the criteria.

When research diagnostic criteria for anorexia nervosa were first
were promulgated at Washington University in the 1970s before they
were modified for inclusion in the Diagnostic and Statistical Manual,
the diagnosis required physiological manifestations that were the result of starvation. Medical and other psychiatric illnesses that could account for weight loss had to be excluded. In the 1980 version of the
American Psychiatric Association criteria (*DSM-III*),[4] weight loss of 25

percent below normal was required; since 1987 (*DSM-III-R*)[5] only 15 percent weight loss is required to make the diagnosis. Quite obviously, if one applied these criteria strictly, more individuals would have been identified as having anorexia nervosa after 1987 than before, even though there was no real change in numbers. Clearly, there is not a sharp line of demarcation between health and illness. A given individual is not healthy at 98 pounds and sick with anorexia nervosa at 97 pounds. Factors other than the precise amount of weight loss enter into the equation. Whether the person is functioning well physiologically and socially is more important than the precise amount of weight that has been lost. A 15 percent weight loss in an overweight person has a different meaning from a 15 percent weight loss in an average weight person. The same proportion of weight loss has yet different significance in a person who was thin initially. Clinical judgment is required to make a rational diagnosis. The state of general health, physiological functioning, prior weight, and the magnitude and rapidity of weight loss are among the variables to be considered.

As the typical adolescent grows and develops, weight tends to increase at a predictable rate. In girls, as a growth chart shows, height tends to increase little after 15 years of age whereas weight continues to increase until age 17 or 18, when it levels off. During mid-adolescence youngsters gain weight at the rate of 10 to 12 pounds per year.

There is great individual variability among people in body build, skeletal structure, and body composition, including lean body mass and fatness. A young girl must have a critical amount of body fat to undergo the changes of puberty, to begin menstruating, and to thrive thereafter. The amount of body fat increases during adolescence— from about 16 percent of total body weight at age 9 to roughly 28 percent by the time a girl's body has fully matured. Menstruation begins when body fat reaches about 24 percent of total body weight.[6] These are averages. There is great variation in these measures from individual to individual. Some girls, particularly short ones, begin menstruating when they weigh as little as 80 pounds; others do not begin to menstruate until they reach 125 pounds or more. The vast majority, however, reach menarche when their weight reaches about 103 pounds. That weight coincides with 24 percent body fat for most.[7] These population norms were arrived at by Rose Frisch and her co-workers at the

Harvard Center for Population Studies. They are highly relevant to our understanding of the endocrine correlates of anorexia nervosa.

The amount of body fat can be estimated during the physical examination using skin fold measurements. Calipers are used to measure the thickness of skin and underlying fat at four specific locations. The sum of these measurements is then converted to the percentage of body fat on a standard table. Anorexic girls who are severely underweight may have as little as 10 percent body fat, or even less.

Another measure that is more meaningful than weight alone is body mass index (BMI). This is derived from height and weight measurements in the metric system.[8]

$$BMI = \text{weight in kg.}/(\text{height in cm})^2$$

The formula can be adapted to the English system of weights and measures:

$$BMI = \text{weight in pounds} \times 703/(\text{height in inches})^2$$

A BMI of 18.5 to 24.9 is considered normal. Twenty-five and greater is considered overweight, and 30 and above obese. Underweight is 18.4 and less; below 15 signifies emaciation. The measure provides a rough indication of whether a person is within an acceptable weight range for her height.

When an individual girl diets and loses weight there is great variability in the consequences, depending on her age, size, and magnitude of weight loss. A 14-year-old girl who loses 10 pounds from 130 pounds to 120 pounds over a two-year period may maintain excellent health and overall adaptation. In contrast, a 12-year-old girl who loses 10 pounds from 100 pounds to 90 pounds could be in serious trouble physiologically, and be ill with anorexia nervosa even though she has lost only 10 percent of her weight. Had she continued to develop normally, she would have weighed 120 pounds at age 14 years. Thus, she would actually be 30 pounds, or 25 percent, below her expected weight at that age. Yet another 13-year-old girl losing the same amount of weight from 110 pounds to 100 pounds might be in a borderline range of weight, still making an acceptable, but tenuous, adaptation.

Tables of "ideal body weight" are not of much use when applied to individuals. One may ask, "Ideal for whom?" These tables imply that healthy weight is to be found within a narrow range. In reality, individuals vary greatly in what constitutes a healthy weight for them. Some are naturally thin, have always been so, and are healthy. I once saw Jody, a junior high school girl, brought by her distressed mother because her health teacher had singled her out, suspecting she had anorexia nervosa. The teacher had become alarmed because Jody's weight was below the 10th percentile for her age and height. By taking a medical history I saw that Jody had always been thin, and other family members were thin. Moreover, she had already had two menstrual periods. She showed no aversion to food, and was eating adequately for continued normal growth. She had not made an effort to diet. She was functioning very well academically and socially. Her mother was reassured that Jody did not have anorexia nervosa.

Obesity has become increasingly frequent and is much more common than anorexia nervosa. It certainly poses health hazards for most, as it increases the risk for heart disease, diabetes, hypertension, and stroke. Better methods for preventing obesity are sorely needed. However, there are some persons of sturdy build who would be considered obese based on the tables. Many of them lead active, healthy lives. Their physiology has adapted to a greater than average weight. Were they to diet to reach their "ideal weight" they would be undernourished and develop symptoms of undernutrition. They would suffer from weakness, fatigue, and in women, from amenorrhea. Humans come in many shapes and sizes. They should not be judged by arbitrary standards. Attempting to fit them all into the same mold is not only unwise but unrealistic.

Remember that an adolescent's growth and development are in a constant state of flux. They do not remain static. Weight changes must therefore be considered in the light of expected development over time. Evaluating the magnitude of an adult's weight loss is easier because weight has normally stabilized by the early twenties.

An intense fear of becoming fat and a disturbance in body image—the psychological criteria that are central to anorexia nervosa—are expressed differently from one person to another. Hilde Bruch, a psychiatrist working at Columbia University in the 1960s and later at Baylor University, was the first person to spend much time listening to the thoughts and feelings of patients with anorexia nervosa. Prior to her work with these patients, psychiatrists tried to discern causes of the disorder, but by and large did not heed the characteristic psychological features that Bruch identified. She described genuine or primary anorexia nervosa as the typical form in which a struggle for control, for a sense of identity, competence, and effectiveness are the main issues.[9] Among these individuals she described three areas of disordered psychological functions. The first is a disturbance in the body image and body concept. The second is a disturbance in the accuracy of the perception or interpretation of stimuli arising in the body, manifested by failure to recognize hunger or satiety. The third outstanding feature is a paralyzing sense of ineffectiveness. Moreover, there is also a strong tendency to be hyperactive and to deny fatigue. Bruch suggested that the core feature among individuals with primary anorexia nervosa is a relentless pursuit of thinness.

Bruch also described an atypical group in which no general picture can be drawn as for the typical cases. She suggested that patients with atypical anorexia nervosa and those with the genuine syndrome look deceptively alike, especially after the condition has existed for some time. In contrast with the typical cases, in whom relentless pursuit of thinness is a key symptom, atypical patients may complain about their weight loss and may not want to stay thin. Some of these patients clearly had emotionally based conflicts or were developing a psychotic illness. In others, depression was the underlying cause.

Long experience has taught me that distinguishing these forms is not always clear-cut. Rather, there is a spectrum of symptoms and a continuum of severity that dictate the treatment. Once weight loss advances to a critical point, the clinical picture that may at first have been atypical resembles the typical form. The psychological features that Bruch suggested as being antecedents of the illness may, in fact, be the result of severe starvation.

In former years it was common for a patient with anorexia nervosa to express the fear of becoming fat. Nowadays that is less common, perhaps because patients are more aware that is expected of them. They may not verbalize this fear, but they express it by failing to gain weight.

Hilde Bruch felt that anorexics had a basic defect in the way they perceived their bodies.[10] This concept has aroused controversy. As with physiological accompaniments of anorexia nervosa, it may be that body image disturbance is a consequence, rather than a precursor, of the disorder. Moreover, it is less common now than in the past for an anorexic patient to say that she thinks she is fat. Marlene, a 17-year-old high school student, markedly underweight, acknowledged that she was too thin and said that she wanted to gain weight. Yet her behavior belied that statement, as she continued to restrict her food intake markedly and avoided the recommendation to eat more.

Amenorrhea, or absence of menstrual periods, is the final criterion for the diagnosis of anorexia nervosa. The requirement that three or more consecutive periods be missed is arbitrary. When weight loss has been rapid, only one or two periods may have been lost, and the individual may clearly be anorexic. Some believe that menstrual periods typically cease as the first sign of anorexia nervosa, before much weight has been lost. They imply that there is an underlying endocrine disorder that triggers the anorexia nervosa. In my experience, the overwhelming majority of girls and women who develop anorexia nervosa lose weight first, and then lose their menstrual periods when a critical amount of weight has been lost. This is consistent with the findings of Rose Frisch, whose studies indicated that menstrual cycles stop with weight loss of 10 percent to 15 percent from the critical weight of 103 pounds, when menstrual periods typically begin.[11] I found that it is valuable to know how much a particular girl weighed when she started menstruating; her periods stop when her weight declines somewhat below that weight. In most instances, the endocrinological disturbances, including the cessation of menses, are consequences of undernutrition with excessive loss of body fat. Premenarchal girls, of course, who develop anorexia nervosa, fail to begin menstruating. The onset of their menses will be delayed as long as they remain significantly underweight. They will remain sexually immature, with a delay of secondary sexual characteristics, including breast development and pubic hair.

All said and done, the formal criteria for diagnosis should not be taken too seriously. They represent the profession's best efforts to codify the characteristics that are observed clinically. They were arrived at by a consensus of experts. Some of the finer points have been changed over the years, but the patients stay the same. When applying the criteria to an individual, the physician needs to maintain perspective and common sense. The responsibility of applying them meaningfully lies in the hands of the physician evaluating the patient.

CHAPTER EIGHT

Disorders That Mimic Anorexia Nervosa

A number of conditions accompanied by weight loss can simulate anorexia nervosa. The most common of these is depression. Another condition that may be difficult to distinguish is inflammatory bowel disease. Also, some endocrine disorders may be misleading. Depression is perhaps most often missed but if the right questions are asked the diagnosis will become clear. Distinguishing these disorders early is important in providing the right treatment quickly.

Depression

Arlene was a 14-year-old girl whose childhood was not unusual. She had close friends with whom she enjoyed socializing at school and talking on the phone in the evening. Recently she and her closest friend had taken up tennis and they hoped to become good enough to try out for her school team. She was a good student with strengths in English and the social sciences. Math was a challenge for her. Her home life was unremarkable, and she felt closer to her mother than to her father. Her parents quarreled occasionally about child rearing, the father believing that the mother was "too soft" on the children. The chief source of conflict at home was Arlene's frequent arguments with her brother, a year younger than she. He had a talent for math and was adept at computers. He frequently let Arlene know that she was "dumb" in math. She complained that he intruded on her space, was a "smart aleck," and was too curious about her belongings.

In the fall her mother noted that Arlene was not the lively, bubbly girl that she had been the previous school year and through the summer. Arlene spent more time by herself in her room and stopped calling her friends. Sometimes she had unexplained crying spells. Her mother became particularly concerned when Arlene became irritable and sarcastic. She discussed these concerns with a friend and concluded that her changed behavior was a part of adolescence, hoping that it would pass. Arlene seemed to be spending more time on her studies, but when her second school report came out, her grades had declined from A's and B's to mostly C's because of incomplete work. This surprised her parents, but they encouraged her to persevere. What concerned her mother even more was that Arlene began picking at her food and frequently said that she wasn't hungry. By the end of November she had actually lost several pounds and began to look thin and haggard. Her mother became alarmed because another student in Arlene's class had recently been diagnosed with anorexia nervosa. She wondered if Arlene was also developing an eating disorder. Arlene was taken to her family physician. She had indeed lost six pounds and was eating very little. He found no physical cause for her weight loss and referred her to me, suspecting she had anorexia nervosa.

In the psychiatric evaluation it became clear that Arlene had no intention to lose weight. She had truly lost her appetite and expressed little interest in food. She did not know the caloric values of foods and had not paid attention to what she was eating. She was not exercising. On the contrary, she found it increasingly hard to attend her tennis lessons and noted that she became exhausted easily when she played. She had lost interest in her activities and schoolwork, finding it hard to keep her mind on her lessons. She had likewise lost interest in being with her friends and could not bring herself to call them as she had in the past. She had some difficulty falling asleep and began to have disturbing dreams. She readily recognized that she was thin and commented that she did not like the bony appearance of her body. When asked if she felt troubled about anything she began to cry, but could not explain just what made her sad.

I recognized that Arlene was depressed and did not have anorexia nervosa. There were no apparent traumatic or precipitating factors to bring on the depression, but it was noted that Arlene's maternal aunt and grandmother had episodes of depression during adolescence from which they recovered without treatment. The grandmother continued to have episodes throughout life during which she withdrew from her family and social contact and took to her bed. Two of these episodes occurred after the birth of her children. Late in life she had a severe depression that required treatment with electroconvulsive therapy.

Depression in adolescence is easily mistaken for anorexia nervosa. The chief difference is that in depression there is true loss of appetite, lack of interest in food, and an absence of intent to lose weight. The magnitude of weight loss is usually much less than in anorexia nervosa. Activity is diminished rather than increased. Depressed mood, manifested by sadness and crying spells, is seen in depression. There may or may not be environmental circumstances that lead to the depression, such as the loss of someone close, a move to a new community, or loss of self-esteem. Most often there is a biological predisposition to develop a depression influenced by heredity.

When anorexia nervosa has been present for a time, symptoms of depression almost invariably intrude. Thus, the conditions superficially may resemble one another. When one inquires about the attitude toward eating and body image, however, the conditions most often are readily distinguished.

Inflammatory Bowel Disease

I was called to see a patient in the hospital who was suspected to have anorexia nervosa. Julia was a 16-year-old girl who had lost 20 pounds over a six-month period, dropping from 125 to 105 pounds. She was lying in her hospital bed, appearing ill and emaciated. Her face was pale, and her arms were thin, showing wasting of her musculature. She complained of abdominal pain and had been unable to eat normal quantities of food. At another clinic she had been diagnosed with anorexia nervosa because of her weight loss, small intake of food, and abdominal pain. She was not yet menstruating. She was referred to us for treatment.

I asked her about the sequence of her symptoms, and she emphasized that they began with abdominal pain, crampy and intermittent in character. She then lost her appetite and was able to eat only small quantities of food. She had no aversion to fattening foods, however. When I asked her whether she had felt fat or was worried about becoming fat, she indicated, on the contrary, that she was distressed about her weight loss. In fact, she wanted to gain weight. She was not constipated but had been having more frequent loose stools than usual.

It became evident that no one had asked her about her attitude about eating and her body image. The assumption was made that she had anorexia nervosa because of her age, lack of menstrual periods, and remarkable weight loss. By asking the right questions, I saw that she did not have anorexia nervosa and sought another cause for her weight loss. Further studies revealed that she had inflammation of her small bowel. The diagnosis of regional ileitis, or Crohn's disease, was made and she was treated by a gastroenterologist. That condition is usually characterized by frequent watery stools, sometimes tinged with blood, and abdominal crampy pain. In Julia's case, diarrhea was not the most prominent feature.

Endocrine Disorders

Salina, a 19-year-old young woman was seen in consultation because of weight loss and agitation. Her mother thought that she had an eating disorder because she was eating large quantities of food and yet losing weight. She suspected that she might be vomiting, although she had no real evidence of this. On examination Salina was restless and agitated, speaking rapidly. She noted that she had the tendency to sweat excessively and said that she could not maintain her weight despite eating frequently. She had no desire to lose weight. Salina's pulse rate was rapid. Laboratory tests confirmed that her metabolic rate was elevated and that her thyroid function was increased. She had hyperthyroidism and was referred to an internist for treatment.

Endocrine disorders, including thyroid disorders and diabetes, are less often mistaken for anorexia nervosa. Patients with *hyperthyroidism*, an *overactive* thyroid gland, have a high level of physical activity not unlike anorexic patients. Their metabolic rate, however, is increased, in contrast with patients with anorexia nervosa, who have a decreased metabolic rate. Hyperthyroid patients perspire excessively, while anorexics have decreased sweating. Hyperthyroid patients also tend to eat excessively. They may lose a moderate amount of weight. *Hypothyroid* patients, those with an *underactive* thyroid gland, resemble anorexic patients in some ways. Their metabolic rate, as in anorexia nervosa, is decreased, and they have decreased sweating. In contrast with anorexic patients they are underactive and do not tend to lose weight.

Patients with diabetes have insulin deficiency and consequently have high blood sugar. At the onset of juvenile diabetes, patients may undergo rapid weight loss. The conditions are not hard to distinguish, however, because there is greatly increased appetite in diabetes. Diabetics also drink excessive quantities of fluids at the onset of their disease. Anorexic patients also may drink excessively, but they restrict their appetite. Those anorexic patients who drink excessively resemble patients with diabetes insipidus, a condition in which antidiuretic hormone is diminished because of a disturbance in the posterior pituitary gland. In anorexia nervosa this same hormone may be diminished as a result of the starvation effect.

Anorexia nervosa and diabetes may coexist. I have seen patients whose insulin requirement was reduced or eliminated temporarily while they were restricting their caloric intake. Thus, their anorexia can mask the diabetes for a time but at the cost of injuring their general health due to their emaciation.

Girls who have never menstruated (primary amenorrhea) and those whose menstrual periods have stopped (secondary amenorrhea) may present a difficult diagnostic challenge. These symptoms occur in anorexia nervosa because of a reduction in gondotrophic hormones and estrogen, which results from starvation. In other conditions failure of the anterior pituitary gland or of the ovaries lead to similar symptoms. Rarely, tumors of the pituitary gland or hypothalamus (part of the brain above the pituitary gland) can resemble anorexia nervosa because the same hormones are affected in each of these conditions. Your daughter's physician may order hormonal studies and imaging studies to distinguish which, if any, of these conditions are present.

CHAPTER NINE

Physiological Effects
of Starvation and Weight Gain

The physiological changes seen in patients with anorexia nervosa are due to undernutrition or semistarvation. *Undernutrition* means inadequate food intake. The term *semistarvation* is used because anorexic patients do not subject themselves to total fasting. Unlike the victims of famine they take in some nourishment. For the most part, the physiological changes of semistarvation are adaptive responses of the body allowing the individual to survive reduced intake of dietary sources of energy. Such adaptations are not without their costs. These costs are impairments that limit the individual's capacity to perform normal physical and mental activities. Semistarvation is associated with energy conservation, adaptations to spare the body's use of glucose and protein while favoring the use of fat, dramatic shifts in fluid and electrolyte balances, and alterations in hypothalamic-pituitary function, leading to amenorrhea and infertility.[1]

When I informed my patients about the effects of starvation, weight loss, and subsequent weight gain, I did so in the following way: When the body is starved it tends to shut down in order to save energy, and it does so in a number of ways. The heart rate drops from a normal rate of 70 or 80 beats per minute to 50 per minute or even less. As a result the blood circulates throughout the body more slowly, causing the hands and feet to become blue and cold. This is most noticeable in the fingertips, with the nail beds often appearing blue, and the fingertips becoming pale or even white in cold weather. This is because the blood is moving sluggishly through the capillaries that are found in the ends of the fingers. When this occurs the red blood cells have become depleted of the oxygen they pick up in the lungs, resulting in the blue, rather than pink appearance of the skin. The blood pressure drops from a level of about 110 mm of mercury, which is a normal reading for a teenage girl, to a level of 90 mm or less. Often the pressure is so low as to be difficult to measure with a sphygmomanometer (blood pressure measuring device). Low blood pressure results in episodes of light-headedness and dizziness, especially when the person stands up quickly or runs up the stairs. That is called orthostatic hypotension (low blood pressure when standing up). Blood pressure can fall low enough to cause a person to pass out or faint. Headaches may occur as well, associated with low blood sugar levels that result from inadequate nourishment.

Weight loss at first causes a depletion of body fat, which is noted when the female shape becomes less curvaceous and more angular in appearance. There a reduction in the size of the breasts, the abdomen, the thighs, and buttocks. It is usually first noticeable in the upper parts of the body, causing the arms and shoulders to become very thin and bony. It is around the shoulders that the collarbones and shoulder blades become sharply apparent. The ribs become more visible, and eventually so do the bones of the hips and pelvis. The body tends at first to use its stored fat for energy when not enough food is taken in for the body's energy needs. Some fat is required for normal health and life. After a considerable amount of body fat is lost, muscle tissue becomes depleted as well, as the body begins to break down muscle cells for energy. This results in ketosis, the accumulation of ketone bodies in the blood, which is a sign of starvation.

When someone first begins dieting, she becomes hungry and must try to ignore the hunger if she doesn't want to eat. If she persists in dieting for weeks on end, however, the feeling of hunger eventually diminishes as the body becomes accustomed to taking in less food. The stomach constricts in size as smaller quantities of food are absorbed. The stomach is a flexible hollow organ made of muscles. The muscles of the stomach wall contract rhythmically to mix food with digestive juices and to break it down in order to digest it. The consistency of the stomach can be compared to a cross between a leather bag, such as the ones the Spaniards use for carrying wine, and a thick rubber balloon. It is shaped much like the wine bags. Highly flexible, it expands or contracts to accommodate almost any amount of food consumed. After a period of undernutrition the stomach progressively shrinks down and assumes a smaller, narrower shape. Then, when a larger meal than usual is eaten, the stomach has to expand, and this causes discomfort as it stretches after having adapted to smaller amounts of food. In a starved person, the capacity of the stomach diminishes, causing it to feel full after even a small amount of food is ingested. Additionally, the amount of time that it takes the stomach to digest a meal and to move the food on to the small intestine increases. The body, in its wisdom, takes longer to digest and to absorb nutrients to derive the maximum benefit from the meager amounts of food ingested.

Liquids pass through the stomach relatively quickly in both normally nourished and undernourished individuals. Solid food normally passes through the stomach within an hour or an hour and a half. In anorexia nervosa, as in other forms of starvation, however, the food may need as long as four to five hours to pass through the stomach. Thus, stomach emptying time for solid food is increased. The slowed emptying of the stomach is the reason a person with anorexia nervosa feels full after eating only a small amount of food, and does not become hungry again for many hours after a meal. This constant feeling of fullness makes it difficult to eat three meals a day. The stomach is still partially full when the next meal comes around. We used to think that the discomfort and bloating after meals was imagined because of the fear of eating and of becoming fat. In actuality, research studies of stomach emptying time have shown that in anorexia nervosa, food remains in the stomach an unusually long time and that the associated discomfort is very real.[2] Many anorexic patients are aware of these feelings, particularly early in the illness. Others seem unaware of feelings of hunger and satiety, especially after the illness has been present for a period of time.

Constipation with small, hard bowel movements accompanies starvation partly because so little food is taken in that there is little to pass as waste. Additionally, because of the increased efficiency with which the body is utilizing the food, most of it is digested and absorbed. Water, from liquids ingested, is absorbed by the intestines. When there is a sudden increase in the amount of food and liquids consumed after a period of starvation, loose, watery stools and diarrhea may occur.

After prolonged starvation, because of changes in sodium and potassium excretion, excessive amounts of fluid may be retained (starvation edema). This is particularly noticeable as swelling of the ankles. When there is rapid re-feeding, sodium is retained and re-feeding edema may occur. Again, this is most noticeable as swelling of the ankles. Swelling of the abdomen and of the face may also appear. Excessive water retention thus can cause rapid increase in weight. This can exert an increased workload on the heart. Even with moderate weight gain there will be some retention of fluids and swelling of the ankles, abdomen, and face. This is not an accumulation of fat and will dissipate in time as healthy eating progresses.

Other physical signs occur when starvation is severe and prolonged. Fine, downy hair, called lanugo, appears on the body. It is similar in appearance to the hair on the body of newborn infants. In anorexic patients it may appear on the face, abdomen, back, or arms. Its color will vary with the hair color and complexion of the individual. It is usually sparse, but at times it may appear quite thick. The mechanism responsible for the growth of this new hair is unknown. When I once mentioned this to a patient of mine, she said, "Oh, we're trying to grow a coat of fur to keep us warm." There may be some truth in that explanation.

The loss of body fat decreases the body's insulation and contributes to anorexics' feeling cold, even in moderately warm weather. They frequently dress in multiple layers of clothing. Slowed circulation of the blood adds to that problem. There are other complications from loss of body fat. In addition to insulating the body, the normal layer of fat beneath the skin serves as protective padding and prevents injuries. Without this protection bones are more likely to break when bumped or put under strain. This risk is aggravated when bones have become weakened and brittle due to decalcification from poor nutrition (osteoporosis).

In some instances, skin color takes on an orange hue, most noticeable on the palms of the hands or soles of the feet and in skin creases inside the elbows. This is caused by high levels of carotene circulating in the blood that become deposited underneath the skin (hypercarotenemia). The color truly is orange and not yellow, as in jaundice.

Nor is it present in the whites of the eyes, where jaundice is detected. It is the pigment that occurs in carrots and other vegetables. It was long assumed that the discoloration was from eating an excess of carrots, which some anorexic patients do, because carrots are so low in calories. Certainly it results when enormous quantities of carrots are eaten, but hypercarotenemia can occur even when carrots are not consumed. The mechanism is a defect in the conversion of ß-carotene to Vitamin A, a process that occurs in the liver. This is one of the differences between the physiological findings in anorexia nervosa and ordinary starvation, but the reason for this remains a puzzle.

Sleep disturbances are common in anorexia nervosa and are probably related to changes in the levels of neurohormones. Early morning awakening is common, as is frequent awakening during the night. Some anorexics stay awake until late into the night, sleeping only a few hours. The reason for the sleep disturbance is a combination of the desire to stay awake to study or exercise, and the endocrine changes that interfere with sleep. During the early stages of starvation the individual may have a false feeling of heightened energy and endurance. Increased levels of adrenalin and other hormones account for this increased level of arousal. It encourages more activity, which burns up excessive calories and leads to further loss of weight, fat, and muscle depletion. One of my patients was so driven to exercise that she monopolized a stair-climbing machine at her local "Y." She began using it three hours daily, day in and day out, despite her extreme emaciation. The staff at the "Y" became so concerned that they barred her from using the facility.

During anorexia nervosa, decreased levels of antidiuretic hormone are produced, resulting in increased output of pale, dilute urine. This resembles a condition called diabetes insipidus, but is actually another result of the hormonal changes due to starvation. It causes increased thirst and excessive fluid intake. It can contribute to frequent night-time awakening as well. When an anorexic person forcibly restricts drinking fluids, as sometimes happens, the opposite occurs. She becomes dehydrated. Urine quantity diminishes and its color darkens. In extreme instances an anorexic patient stops drinking almost entirely, even spitting out her saliva rather than swallowing it. I have seen this relatively more frequently in boys than in girls.

Menstrual periods stop after a certain amount of weight has been lost. In girls who have not yet had their first period, the onset of menses is delayed. There is controversy in the literature about the time when periods cease among individuals with anorexia nervosa. Several studies report that menstrual periods cease first, before much weight is lost. That has not been my observation in teenage girls who develop anorexia nervosa. Almost invariably, they lose weight first, and when their weight falls below a critical level, which is unique for each, the periods stop.

Typically the person with anorexia nervosa is relatively dehydrated. As she begins eating a bit more with the initial meal plan, her body will retain a certain amount of water. This may cause a weight increase of a pound or two, and may be frightening to the patient. Next, the body retains and stores glycogen, a readily convertible source of energy, in the muscles and the liver. This may add another half pound of weight. For the first week or two, weight hopefully will stabilize, if the prescribed diet is consumed, and a small amount of weight is retained, from water and glycogen. Only after that has occurred and the diet has become better balanced is any fat deposited in the body. This may begin to happen after about three weeks of weight gain. Fat is necessary for survival and serves the several purposes mentioned earlier. When one gains weight, it is deposited in a thin layer all over the body, where it serves as protective padding and insulation. A certain amount of fat is also necessary for the female body to produce the hormones needed for menstruation and fertility. Several pounds of fat distributed all over the body are hardly visible. More disturbing to the anorexic patient is the weight gain caused by water retention because it can be seen as swelling in the face, over the abdomen, and in other parts of the body. The anorexic girl often thinks this is fat. Gradually the body begins to fill out sunken cheeks and the hollows between the bones visible in the shoulders and between the ribs. Eventually, the buttocks, hips, and thighs will begin to fill in, and the breasts will increase in size. Muscle tissue also is repaired and develops in mass and weight. As sufficient nourishment is taken in, a moderate increase in exercise should accompany it. This will build muscle and increase strength.

Contrary to the hope and desire of many, we cannot selectively determine where to take off weight when we are dieting, nor can we determine where to put it on when we are gaining weight. Unfortunately, genetics determines your body shape and size, and control this. Thin figures or rotund figures have been valued at different times in history and in different cultures. Depending on your point of view, you may feel fortunate to have a naturally thin and angular figure like that of Twiggy, the famous British model of the 1960s who was revered as the ideal when the anorexic figure became popular. Middle Easterners, however, value a different shape. A story was once circulated that an Arab sheik made a marriage proposal to Brooke Shields, with whose beauty he was very much taken when he saw her on movie location in Saudi Arabia. He stipulated, however, that she must gain at least 30 pounds to become his bride. She declined the offer.

Each anorexic girl needs to learn what constitutes a healthy weight for herself and come to accept her natural body shape and size. She needs to learn to see herself realistically, as others do. Ultimately she should value attributes beyond her physical appearance. Unfortunately, our society sends the wrong messages to our children—that beauty and good looks are the most desirable values. This is perpetuated for young women of all ages, from baby contests to the Miss America Pageant. Parents and teachers should try to counter these influences by instilling in children the sense that their worth is measured by the values that they learn and by the skills that they attain rather than by their external looks. The burden of accomplishing this falls on individual parents, teachers, and therapists for I am not optimistic that society will soon change its message. Images seen in magazines, in the movies, and on television are too much influenced by the advertising industry to change.

CHAPTER TEN

How Is Fertility Affected?

"You may recover from anorexia nervosa, but you'll never bear children," is what many patients are told by their physicians. True enough, the disease profoundly affects the sex hormones and the reproductive system in both females and males. Impairment of endocrine function is signaled by amenorrhea in girls. Youngsters of both genders lose their sexual interest when they have anorexia nervosa. Figure 7 shows the interrelationships among pituitary, adrenal, and gonadal hormones. Starvation influences the hypothalmus in the brain, which controls the anterior pituitary gland. The anterior pituitary, the "master" gland, affects the other endocrine organs. The levels of pituitary hormones are diminished and, in turn, cause reduction in estrogen levels in females and testosterone in males. The system reverts to its prepubertal state, resulting in the sex life of a 9-year-old housed in the body of a 15-year-old. Among adolescent girls with anorexia nervosa, ultrasound studies of the ovaries have shown that the ovaries remain small and undeveloped.[1,2] The sexual feelings and urges of adolescence are put on hold. In anorexia nervosa the pituitary-adrenal-gonadal axis is suppressed. It may remain that way for many years. Some anorexic patients, indeed, maintain a chronically undernourished state. Consequently they never are able to have children. Their sex organs have atrophied and remain inactive. This tends to occur among those anorexics who have lost the greatest amount of weight and those who remain undernourished for the longest periods of time. Such women

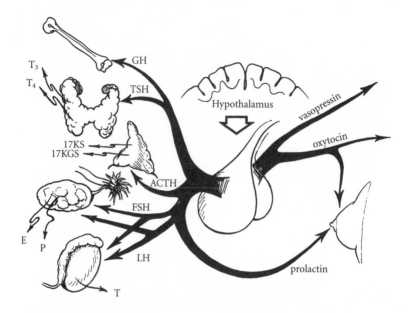

Figure 7. Hypothalamic-pituitary-end organ relationships showing hormones that are affected in anorexia nervosa. From Lucas, AR, Anorexia nervosa: historical background and biopsychosocial determinants, Seminars in Adolescent Med, 1986; 2:5. ACTH, adrenocorticotropic hormone; E, estrogen; FSH, follicle-stimulating hormone; GH, growth hormone; 17-KGS, 17-ketogenic steroid; 17-KS, 17-ketosteroid; LH, luteinizing hormone; P, progesterone; T, testosterone, T_3, triiodothyronine, T_4 thyroxine; TSH, thyroid-stimulating hormone.

become emaciated hollow shells with cadaver-like faces, their sallow skin drawn tightly over their fragile bones. They may be vocationally productive, busily engaged in a whirlwind of activity, but they lead lonely, isolated lives devoid of intimate human contact.

Fortunately, that is not the inevitable outcome. Nor is it the usual outcome. A much more favorable course is the rule rather than the exception. The ultrasound studies show that with weight recovery the ovaries develop normally. Most individuals recover from their illness. Menstrual periods return, signaling the restoration of endocrine function. The time sequence most often is restoration of weight to normal levels, dissipation of abnormal thoughts about food and appearance, and the return of menses. Then the person is emotionally and physically prepared for procreation. There are exceptions to the sequence. The gradual steps may be telescoped in time, with pregnancy occurring before the capacity for fertility is announced by menstruation. Such was the story of Bonnie, who married and became pregnant following recovery from anorexia nervosa without having resumed her menstrual periods.

Shana had severe anorexia nervosa during her teens. She continued to be very thin, pallid, and fragile looking throughout her early adult life. Never very confident in herself, she worked diligently on her studies, devoting unusually long hours to the material that her peers seemed to master much more quickly. She was tense and fastidious and self-critical of her achievement. She had felt dominated by a father whom she thought she could never sufficiently please. After years of study, interrupted by periods of treatment and hospitalization for anorexia nervosa, she became an attorney. Law school was a struggle for her because she had not recovered from her undernourished state. Unlike her aggressive colleagues she was quite unassertive and introverted. Yet once she completed law school she seemed to come into her own. She was sensitive to the needs of others and was very empathic toward her clients, especially troubled adolescents who had run afoul of the law. She went out of her way devoting extra time and efforts to counseling these youngsters. It seemed that a strong maternal instinct drove her to take a special interest in these clients. Her profession consumed her interest and her time. As a young adult, when she was undernourished, she had little inclination for dating. It seemed unlikely that she would ever marry or have children of her own. Remarkably, though, in her late twenties she had gained weight, married, and became a mother. The fertility that she demonstrated in the ensuing years was even more surprising. At last count she had produced a child every year for seven years. Shana had become a healthy, robust mother who had come into her own physically, matrimonially, and professionally. Once she had achieved her goal of being a lawyer and was gratified by having grateful clients who admired her, she found the freedom to relax. No longer did she need to compete for grades and academic achievement. She had become confident in herself and no longer needed to prove her worth. Shana's case is atypical but amply illustrates that anorexia nervosa need not obviate eventual fertility.

In our community study, based on patients representing the broad range of severity of anorexia nervosa, there was much variability in fertility. Some never married and were childless. However, the women who recovered from anorexia nervosa had as many as six children. One man with a history of anorexia nervosa fathered seven children. Most had fewer children but had regained their fertility.[3]

Psychiatrists see a skewed population of patients, including the most severe cases of anorexia nervosa. They see those who have not recovered, including those who have lost their fertility. Gynecologists, on the other hand, see a broader spectrum of patients, including many healthy women. Frequently they are asked to see young women who have missed their menstrual periods. Among those are a sizable number of individuals with early signs of anorexia nervosa. Some gynecologists are loath to make that diagnosis, feeling the label will stigmatize the patient. Dr. Elizabeth Mussey, a wise and compassionate gynecologist who retired from Mayo Clinic many years ago, never wrote the diagnosis of anorexia nervosa in the medical records of the many young women whom she saw with the disorder.[4] She signed out the charts with the diagnosis "hypothalamic amenorrhea." When I read these charts, the familiar story was all there. Typically, the patient would be an older teenage girl who had missed several menstrual periods. She had also lost weight, and Dr. Mussey would carefully have documented a history of inappropriate dieting preceding the onset of the loss of menstrual periods. Quite often there would be a comment about how the girl was afraid of becoming fat. The medical evaluation determined that there was no endocrinological disease underlying the amenorrhea. The hypothalamic hormones that activate the anterior pituitary gland, and consequently the ovaries, were reduced. The girl and her parents would be reassured that she did not have an endocrine illness causing her menstrual failure. The treatment recommendations would be to gain sufficient weight so that the periods could resume. More often than not the result would be salutary.

Gynecologists Starkey and Lee obtained follow-up data on 58 women with anorexia nervosa seen at Mayo Clinic to determine how many of them became fertile after their illness.[5] Forty-one amenorrheic women had recovered as indicated by satisfactory weight gain. In 38, regular menses resumed after three months to several years. Twenty-eight of them tried to become pregnant, and all but one conceived.

Janelle weighed only 76 pounds in her early 20s. She had no menstrual periods during that time. She was married and gained a little weight, just enough for her menstrual periods to return. She became pregnant but remained underweight, eating sparingly throughout the pregnancy. The greatest weight she reached during her pregnancy was only 86 pounds. Nonetheless, she delivered a healthy, full-term, baby boy, who was normal in weight, when she was 26 years old. Following delivery her weight fell again to 76 pounds. Her case illustrates that, on rare occasions, pregnancy can occur even in the undernourished state. Janelle's experience is an exception, most definitely not to be recommended. Her child was very fortunate to be normal. More often maternal malnutrition affects the birth weight, development, and intelligence of the infant. Having a baby in such a severely undernourished state greatly increases the risks of pregnancy, both to the infant and to the mother. Janelle continued to starve herself, and several years later she weighed only 70 pounds and was consuming only 500 calories per day. Her 3-year-old son, however, was thriving. Janelle was nourishing him well but sadly neglecting her own nutrition.

Russell and others have written of the risks to babies whose mothers have anorexia nervosa.[6] The babies may be born undernourished. The mothers may become even more undernourished. Some underfeed their infants, and these children were found to have suffered food deprivation with severe reduction in weight and height for age. However, catch-up growth was possible. While the women who were reported in this study deprived their children of food, other women who have had anorexia nervosa may inappropriately overfeed their infants out of their own distorted nutritional convictions.

The ability to become fertile and to bear children after anorexia nervosa varies tremendously from person to person. Almost anything is possible. The sooner that good nutrition and menstruation are restored, the more likely it is that fertility will resume. However, in some cases menstruation may have ceased for years before it is restored. At the onset of the illness or during its acute course it is impossible to make predictions about the eventual fertility outcome. For those who hope to have children, the wisest course is to resume normal eating habits as soon as possible and to achieve a healthy weight that will allow the generative processes to flourish.

CHAPTER ELEVEN

Bulimia, Bulimia Nervosa, and Binge Eating

Nora was a very pretty girl, the only child and heiress to a sizable lumber fortune. Her family lived in the Pacific Northwest. Her father had died of liver failure due to chronic alcoholism while she was still in her teens. Her mother was a slender beauty whom Nora much admired. Nora, at 5' 3", had matured quite early, weighing 123 pounds when she was 12. After she went away to boarding school at age 15 she was quite chubby and compared herself unfavorably with her peers, and so she began to diet. Quite rapidly her weight dropped to below 100 pounds. But she was unable to maintain her diet. By the time she was 18 she weighed 130 pounds. After graduating from boarding school she renewed her effort to lose weight. Her mother became increasingly concerned about Nora's refusal to eat regular meals, but Nora insisted that she was fine and wanted to be left alone. Her physician found no illness to account for her weight loss and recommended more rest and appetizing food. While she had all the hallmarks of anorexia nervosa, that diagnosis was never made. Her mother decided to take her on a cruise around the world, thinking that the change in scenery, fresh ocean air, and the availability of plentiful appealing food would improve Nora's appetite. This was not to be. Nora shunned the lavish cuisine served frequently throughout the day and evening and continued losing even more weight on the cruise. Photographs showed her as a pitifully emaciated young woman against the backdrop of an artfully picturesque buffet. She returned home and began college, all the time becoming increasingly undernourished. By the time she was 24 she weighed only 72 pounds. Rather suddenly, after years of self-starvation, Nora began to experience food craving that she could no longer resist. She became greatly distressed because she would eat everything she could get her hands on. Her weight rapidly increased, but she was still abnormally thin at 94 pounds when she came to see me.

Nora's distress stemmed from her inability to stop her intense craving for food and her voracious hunger. Food had become an almost constant preoccupation for her. She had not sought treatment for being underweight but now was desperate for help. Her body was still very thin but her cheeks had a swollen "chipmunk" appearance. She described having eating binges every two to three weeks when she would gorge herself. If nothing else was available she would even eat unthawed food from her freezer. At times she would empty a vending machine of candy bars and consume them all. She never made herself vomit but ate to the point of abdominal distention and exhaustion, when she would collapse and go to sleep with a severe stomachache. These binges would make her weight rise as much as 8 to 10 pounds in a single day. After these binges she would starve herself for days.

Cassie was a 15-year-old girl who was seen because of depression. She had begun to have disturbing dreams of dying and was afraid she would harm herself after the death of a close friend. She was quite normal in weight and had no signs of an eating disorder. When she came to her appointment the day after Thanksgiving both of her eyes were severely bloodshot with extensive hemorrhages in the whites. When I asked her about them she said she had rubbed her eyes because they felt irritated as if something were in them. The bleeding was beneath the conjunctivae, the transparent membranes that cover the whites of the eyes. It did not extend into the pupils. This is known as a subconjunctival hemorrhage. I suspected that there was another cause than local irritation. Later she confided to her school counselor that she had overeaten at Thanksgiving dinner and secretly made herself vomit. She found it difficult to do so. She gagged herself, at first without success. Then she strained and retched until she regurgitated much of her dinner. Afterward she noted that her eyes were filled with blood. Within two weeks her eyes had healed. Although she was careful in subsequent weeks to avoid vomiting, several months later she overate again and induced vomiting more easily and without incurring the ocular hemorrhages. Her vomiting became habitual. Whenever she felt she had overeaten, she made herself vomit. Her weight, however, remained in the normal range, never varying more than a few pounds.

A much more devastating form of bingeing and purging was experienced by Arla. She had anorexia nervosa as a teenager, from which she made a partial weight recovery with hospital treatment using a behavioral approach. She persisted in her fear of fatness, however, after leaving the hospital. Relentlessly she strove to be thin. For a number of years she succeeded in restricting her eating, but eventually she began overeating on occasion. Episodes of eating binges grew more frequent and the quantity of food she consumed increased as well. Arla resorted to diet pills, vomiting, enemas, and abusing laxatives in order to avoid gaining weight. Vomiting came easily to her and she experienced a sense of elation when she emptied her stomach. After a large meal she would take quantities of laxatives. Purging made her feel empty and pure. Enema use became habitual. She had ceased to have menstrual periods. Her teeth became eroded from frequent vomiting as the acid from her stomach wore off her tooth enamel. The damage was so severe she had to have most of her teeth capped by the time she was 20. Her blood potassium level frequently became so low that there was concern she would sustain damage to her kidneys and heart. She had extensive treatment, both in hospitals and as an outpatient. This included individual psychotherapy and family therapy. Nonetheless, her condition did not improve. She had become depressed over her inability to control her eating and took an aspirin overdose in an attempt to kill herself. She reached her lowest weight of 63 pounds at age 19. Her eating habits had become completely deranged when she came to see me at the age of 21. She exercised compulsively and frantically. At 5'5" she weighed 103 pounds. She was highly motivated to overcome her inability to control her eating. Yet she still felt fat and hoped to weigh 90 pounds.

This book would be incomplete without mentioning the eating disorders that are the flip side of anorexia nervosa. A full discussion of these disorders could take up an entire volume, but because there is such a close relationship between them and anorexia nervosa, they are considered here. Some patients have anorexia nervosa in its purely restricting form while many develop a mixture of symptoms that include binge eating and purging.

Strictly speaking, bulimia means "ox hunger," voracious appetite, or an abnormal constant craving for food. The widespread recognition of eating disorders during the past 20 or 30 years has caused the term to become distorted. Most persons who use the word bulimia now think of it as being synonymous with self-induced vomiting. Recent editions of Webster's Dictionary include in its definition that it is a serious eating disorder characterized by compulsive overeating usually followed by self-induced vomiting or laxative or diuretic abuse. Gerald Russell at the Institute of Psychiatry in London first described bulimia nervosa in 1979 as an ominous variant of anorexia nervosa.[1] He had observed women who at first had anorexia nervosa and then after some time began binge eating and purging. Purging most often is done by self-induced vomiting or by using laxatives to rid oneself of unwanted food. We do not know whether bulimia nervosa is really a new disease or whether it existed unrecognized in the past. I suspect that it occurred in the past, but not with the frequency we now encounter. We do know that it became more common in the 1980s and then surpassed anorexia nervosa in frequency. Timothy Soundy and I identified 103 residents of Rochester, Minnesota, who fulfilled diagnostic criteria for bulimia nervosa during the period from 1980 to 1990. One hundred of these were women and only three were men. The incidence (number of new cases) in females rose sharply from 7 per 100,000 persons in 1980 to 50 per 100,000 persons in 1983, and then remained relatively constant at around 30 per year (see Figure 4, page 26).[2] Kenneth Kendler and his co-workers at the Virginia Institute for Psychiatric and Behavioral Genetics in Richmond, using genetic epidemiological twin-study techniques, established that 1 in 25 women is at risk for developing the syndrome of bulimia nervosa at some time during her life.[3]

Undoubtedly Russell's identification of the syndrome led to its increasing recognition by physicians during the 1980s. It is also likely that there has been a real increase in its occurrence during recent times. Only a small proportion of individuals with bulimia nervosa are in treatment or have been identified. It has been estimated that perhaps only a third of cases are recognized.[4] The vast majority of those who practice bulimic behaviors do so infrequently and give them up before the behaviors cause great harm to their health. Others, however, distressed by every pound that they gain, become so obsessed by the behaviors that they can no longer stop. These are the people who suffer serious health complications. They may even die of their disease.

The bulimic disorders vary greatly in their severity and longevity, and in the harm that they do. It is common among college women to "pig out" on weekends and to force themselves to vomit afterward.[5] Surveys of college students found that a surprisingly high percentage, even more than half of the women, have binged and vomited on occasion. Fewer men have done so, and voluntary vomiting is rare among them. The vast majority of women who indulge in vomiting see its futility and give it up in short order. Many of them come to realize the potential harm they do to their health. A smaller number continue their unsavory behavior and use it as a means of weight control. Their weight fluctuates from day to day and from week to week, but they do not become excessively thin or overweight. They may begin to take diet pills, laxatives, and diuretics to prevent weight gain. Eventually these harmful behaviors take their toll because of excessive loss of water and electrolytes, particularly potassium. This can lead to disturbances in heart and kidney functioning. The harmful behaviors may remain hidden for a long time before health becomes compromised.

Anorexia nervosa, once it is established, is easy to recognize because the individual has become so thin. Bulimia nervosa and its variants may remain hidden because weight remains largely within the normal range. To be sure, it may fluctuate considerably—as much as 10 or 12 pounds in a single day—because the body retains a large quantity of fluid after a binge, but this is then eliminated by purging. It is not unusual for those who engage in these dangerous behaviors to take large quantities of diuretics and laxatives to get rid of body fluid. There are clues that may be observed by family members or by friends. These include the unexplained disappearance of food, such as cookies or other baked goods, frequent trips to the bathroom immediately after meals, and changes in physical appearance. Severe binge eating results in puffiness that may be visible in the face, particularly around the eyes and in the cheeks, and in swelling of the abdomen and of the ankles. When episodic gorging has continued for a long time, the glands that produce saliva become overactive and swollen. They are located in the cheeks, under the angles of the jaw, and underneath the chin. This swelling gives the face a "chipmunk" appearance.

Anorexia nervosa occurs most frequently during mid-adolescence. The bulimic disorders occur somewhat later, most frequently during the 20s. Even more so than anorexia nervosa, they are vastly more common in women than in men. While it is not uncommon for men to have eating binges, often accompanied by alcohol consumption, men do not worry as much as women about the weight they put on as a consequence. On the contrary, among some groups of men, a sizable beer belly is even a status symbol.

The most serious form of bulimia nervosa begins in people who first have anorexia nervosa. Typically their undernourished state has persisted for a year or more. They reach the point at which they can no longer exert full control over their hunger in order to maintain their meager diets. In other words, they become overwhelmed by the hunger that they have suppressed so long. They give in to their biological need and indulge in cravings they have long avoided. They discover that they are able to vomit what they ate and are relieved when they succeed in doing so. Learning to induce vomiting may be difficult at first if they do not have a ready gag reflex. They may have to work at trying to gag themselves with their finger or with a spoon. In time, vomiting becomes easier and they feel more free to eat favored food, even to binge on large quantities because they know they can get rid of it. One patient told me that she had learned to "have my cake and eat it too." As self-induced vomiting becomes habitual, many patients learn that they do not have to gag themselves. They simply bend over or push on their abdomens. Syrup of ipecac causes vomiting, intended as an antidote for accidental poisoning. Some bulimic patients have used it to induce vomiting. When taken frequently or in large quantities it is highly dangerous because of the damage it causes to the heart muscle.

A tell-tale sign of self-induced vomiting is calluses over the knuckles from abrading them against the upper incisor teeth while sticking the fingers down the throat. This is known as Russell's sign or "bulimia blisters."[6] Another physical sign of vomiting is erosion of the dental enamel. This is at first apparent to dentists who examine the teeth during a routine visit. It may become severe and widespread, leading to dental caries when the protective enamel has worn away. It is caused by the action of stomach acid on the hard enamel surfaces. I have seen patients with such extensive tooth decay that their teeth have to be capped or extracted.

In the worst cases a vicious circle evolves in which binge eating and purging occurs many times a day. There is loss of control over eating, which was so valued in the early phase of anorexia nervosa, and guilt about excessive eating. Purging may be induced simply by vomiting, or complicated by the use of laxatives and enemas. The purging gives an immediate sense of relief associated with the feeling of emptiness. However, this is followed by a sense of guilt and recrimination because patients know it is the wrong thing to do. Patients with bulimia nervosa often have impulsive behaviors aside from their eating. They may resort to shoplifting or stealing money in order to buy food.

Binges may involve huge amounts of food. Some people only binge and never vomit. They eat until their stomachs feel as though they will burst. Some bingers have reported eating 5000 calories at a single sitting. The stomach can expand to an enormous size; only very rarely there have been reports of the stomach rupturing.

The *Diagnostic and Statistical Manual of Mental Disorders* (*DSM-IV*) lists two forms of bulimia nervosa; the purging type and the nonpurging type. In general, bulimia nervosa is characterized by recurrent episodes of binge eating, recurrent inappropriate compensatory behavior to prevent weight gain, and undue concern over one's body shape and weight. An episode of binge eating is defined as eating an amount of food that is definitely larger than most people would eat during a similar period of time. It also implies a lack of control over eating during the episode, such as the feeling that one cannot stop eating or control what or how much one is eating. Inappropriate compensatory behaviors to prevent weight gain include self-induced vomiting; misuse of enemas; misuse of laxatives, diuretics, or other medications; fasting; or excessive exercise. In the purging type the individual has regularly engaged in self-induced vomiting or the misuse of laxatives, diuretics, or enemas. In the nonpurging type the individual has used other inappropriate compensatory behaviors, such as fasting or excessive exercise, but has not engaged in self-induced vomiting or the misuse of laxatives, diuretics, or enemas.[7]

I believe that most patients who are said to die of anorexia nervosa have developed bulimia nervosa and die of complications related to electrolyte problems, quite often related to laxative and diuretic abuse. Dying of starvation is extremely rare in this day and age. Karen Carpenter, the renowned singer, received much publicity when she suffered from anorexia nervosa. She was shown on magazine covers in a grossly emaciated state. The actual cause of her death was not reported.

In recent years binge eating disorder has been described as a condition in which the consumption of large quantities of food was not followed by purging. There is controversy about whether this should be considered a disorder or merely a variation of normal eating. Quite obviously, the quantity of food consumed and the frequency with which the overeating occurs must be considered in determining whether the behavior is unhealthy and abnormal. Some persons who engage in bingeing do so infrequently and its practice does not lead to an increase in weight. Others gain weight over time and become obese.

The *Diagnostic and Statistical Manual* defines binge-eating disorder as a condition characterized by recurrent episodes of binge eating. Marked distress accompanies the episodes, and they are not associated with the use of compensatory behaviors (purging, fasting, or excessive exercise). Individuals who engage in binge eating eat more than most people would eat under similar circumstances, they eat more rapidly, eat when they don't feel hungry, or feel disgusted with themselves after overeating. The disorder has not achieved recognition as an "official diagnosis" in the *Manual* but is listed in an appendix as a new category that is under study.[8]

Bulimic disorders vary greatly in their form and consequences. At one end of the spectrum they are mild or transient and blend in with normal variations in eating habits. At the other end they are serious life-threatening illnesses. They can begin in undernourished individuals who have anorexia nervosa. More commonly they occur in those who have never been underweight but who are struggling to avoid becoming fat. Binge eaters may maintain normal weight if their indiscretions are infrequent or if they restrain their eating between binges. Many, however, become obese.

CHAPTER TWELVE

Treatment

The treatment of patients with anorexia nervosa is both a science and an art. The science deals with the physical aspects that resulted from undernutrition, and the art deals with the person in whom the disorder exists. Anorexic patients must change their eating patterns to improve their nutrition and to restore an appropriate weight. Dealing with the unique personalities of patients is largely an art; they must be understood for the individuals they are. This is why the sensitivity of the therapist is paramount in determining whether a working relationship will be established between patient and therapist.

Amy had begun her diet in her fourteenth year after a schoolmate commented that her hips were getting fat. She was rapidly undergoing pubertal changes and had gained 10 pounds the previous year to reach 112 pounds. But within six months, she lost 20 percent of her body weight and dropped to 89 pounds. At that weight she looked very thin but not emaciated. Two months earlier her family physician had made the diagnosis of anorexia nervosa and had advised her to gain weight. Nonetheless, she continued to lose. Her parents brought Amy to me to confirm the diagnosis and to treat her. They complained that she had become very stubborn, a marked change from her previously compliant and conforming demeanor. Whenever they confronted her and urged her to eat, she shed tears and ran to her room. Mealtimes had become a frequent battleground. During her first interview with me Amy protested that she was fat and she hated her flabby thighs. She was animated and vivacious and readily talked about her wish to be accepted by a group of popular girls in her school. Although she had always respected her parents, she complained that they were bugging her about eating. She wanted to make her own decisions about what she ate. I listened to her at length and then told her that her parents and her family doctor were concerned that she was harming her health. I told her that I would evaluate the situation and then would give her my opinion. In answer to specific questions she noted that she felt cold much of the time, that some of her hair was falling out, and that she found it harder to concentrate on her schoolwork. Her menstrual periods, which had begun a year earlier, had stopped. I weighed and measured her and examined her. She was thin, having very little fat tissue on her body. Her hands were cold and blue. Her shoulders and upper arms, particularly, appeared wasted, signaling recent weight loss.

I spent some time describing my findings to her, explaining that she showed definite signs of undernourishment. On a growth chart I showed her that girls of her age usually gained 10 or 12 pounds a year until they stopped growing. She was still growing in height, having become an inch-and-a-half taller during the past year. I explained that she had become seriously undernourished and that her health and ability to function effectively had become impaired. I told her that she might disagree with me but I knew that in order for her to be healthy and to grow up she would have to regain some of the weight she had lost. This would mean, first of all, to stop losing weight, and then gradually to begin gaining some weight as her body matured and continued to grow. She acknowledged that she did want to grow up, that she wanted her menstrual periods to come back because she wanted children some day. She also noted that her breasts had stopped developing. I asked Amy to estimate the width of her waist, her hips, and her "stomach" (abdomen), front to back, by holding out her two hands. Her estimates were about 50 percent greater than her actual measurements. She particularly overestimated the size of her stomach. This came as a surprise to her and demonstrated that she imagined herself as much bigger than she really was. I asked her to describe in general what she ate each day. As expected, the amounts were woefully inadequate. I told her that she would need to come back weekly and we would talk about her feelings about herself, her fears about becoming fat, her conflicts with her parents, and her relationships with her peers. I would want her to see the dietitian I worked with in order to find out more accurately just how much she was eating. In preparation for this visit I asked her to write down what she ate the next several days. The dietitian would discuss her nutritional needs and prescribe a meal plan designed at first to stop weight loss and then to increase her weight gradually. I explained that it would be difficult for her to make this change, and that she would feel too full after each meal. She might become very anxious, even panicky, about how she felt after eating. Nonetheless, this was necessary for her to get well.

I met with Amy's parents and explained much of what I had found and recommended. I advised them to let Amy know how much they were concerned but to stop admonishing her to eat. That would only lead to more arguments and resistance. They should leave the expectation for eating appropriately to the dietitian and to me. Being forthright and direct with Amy assured her that I would be open and honest with her. She also saw that she would be listened to. We would advise her, based on our medical knowledge, as to how much food she needed to eat, but she would be in control of carrying out our plan.

The initial interview with Amy took two hours and I spent an additional half-hour with the parents. Amy did not want to change her eating habits, but she acknowledged that she wanted to be healthy. She listened with interest when I told her about the physiological effects of undernutrition, although she still believed that she was not undernourished. To confirm this she pointed out the "healthy" foods, including fruits and vegetables, that she was eating. It seemed to hit home to her, though, that her feeling cold and her inability to concentrate in school were signs that all was not well. I explained to her that her metabolism had slowed down in order to conserve energy. Seeing the dietitian reinforced many of the concepts that I had raised with Amy. The dietitian was nonjudgmental, reviewed Amy's food records, and laid out a plan that would at first aim to stop weight loss, and then gradually to increase weight.

Amy agreed to keep daily food records and to weigh and record all of the foods she ate. This would assure her that she would not eat too much (her greatest fear), and yet would also assure us that she ate the necessary amounts (which would be difficult). By the end of the second week she actually lost almost two more pounds, although there were days when she gained a half-pound or a pound. Those days were agonizing to Amy. It took a great deal of assurance from us to convince Amy that she would not gain a pound every day and that she would not continue to gain indefinitely on the small meal plan that we prescribed. To gain anything and to keep that weight on, she would need to increase the daily amounts from time to time. By the third week her weight stabilized, and by the fourth week she had actually gained. She became more accustomed to the feeling of fullness after meals. She needed much assurance that the bulge she noted over her stomach was not fat, but simply her stomach stretching to contain the modest amount of food that she ingested. One evening she telephoned in tears because her stomach felt "so fat." I reminded her that in her undernourished state the food that she ate actually stayed in her stomach for a very long time, but this would gradually improve as her nutrition and health got better. Despite feeling too full, she would need to continue eating the prescribed amounts.

Regular sessions with the dietitian were an important part of the treatment. A meal plan was designed and the dietitian supervised its gradual progression. Education about healthy eating habits was the goal.

Amy was able to follow our recommendations quite faithfully. There were some setbacks, but they were overcome. Within six months she had regained the weight that she had lost, and in another six months she was continuing to grow and gain at the expected rate for her age. Almost from the beginning of treatment she was eager to talk about her struggles with her parents, and particularly about her interactions with her peers at school. Rather than focusing too much on the past, I encouraged her to talk about her hopes and aspirations for the future. The appointments were gradually decreased in frequency from once a week to once a month near the end of the year that the dietitian and I worked with her. I had kept a weight chart for Amy to see. On it I recorded her weight at each appointment. When she did consistently well for a period of time, and when she achieved certain goals, I gave her a colorful sticker as a reward. These stickers said, "Good job" or "Excellent," and kept treatment in a light vein. Though she was 14 years old, Amy appreciated this recognition with some pride. Gradually my goal for improved nutrition also became her own. Amy felt free to eat foods she had long avoided, and little by little she was guided more by her hunger than by her fears. She reached the point at which she no longer needed to think about her meal plan but could again eat spontaneously.

Amy began telling me that she had become alienated from her friends who were "boy crazy" and from some who were taking drugs. Their actions bothered her, yet she wanted to be accepted by them. Much of her self-derogatory attitude was focused on her physical appearance. We discussed ways of seeking friends who shared her values and who would appreciate her for who she was. By focusing on her abilities and improving her social skills she was able to be less preoccupied with her negative self-image.

I met with the parents from time to time to discuss their concerns. Her mother could understand Amy's concerns about her body shape, but her father found it difficult to fathom how a healthy young girl could starve herself. They had many questions, but grew less anxious about Amy as they saw the positive changes in her behavior.

Amy's positive response to treatment was perhaps atypical, but it was by no means unusual. She showed less vehement resistance to treatment and was able to engage in a cooperative relationship more easily than most. She was fortunate to enter treatment quite early before the disease and its starvation effects had become deeply ingrained. The conflictual interaction that had evolved with her parents was fairly quickly interrupted. They had a strong bond that superseded the discord that occurred after Amy began dieting excessively.

Treatment all too often is much more difficult and protracted as evidenced by the story of Enid, who needed hospitalization because of her severely undernourished state and her adamant unwillingness to cooperate with treatment. Enid had had several hospitalizations for treatment of anorexia nervosa in another state after she was diagnosed at the age of 16. In treatment programs that enforced high caloric meals using behavioral therapy, she regained some of her weight while in the hospital. In these programs daily weight gain was rewarded by increased privileges. When she lost weight some privileges were withdrawn. She did not intend to maintain this weight but went along with the expectations in order to get out of the hospital. Each time she left the hospital her weight rapidly declined again. Outpatient treatment was attempted next. She saw a therapist whose orientation was to explore Enid's past and to make interpretations about her psyche. Family therapy focused on early childhood problems and her hostile interaction with her parents. The therapist felt that Enid's emotional problems and her conflicted family life needed to be addressed first, before her disturbed eating could be dealt with. More than a year of therapy went by, but Enid's increasingly bizarre eating habits became even more firmly entrenched. Addressing her family problems did not resolve her eating disorder. On the contrary, she became increasingly alienated from her family as she and they blamed each other for her illness. Her weight had dropped to a dangerously low level, and Enid had begun episodes of binge eating, after which she would make herself vomit. Hospitalization was recommended again, but she refused. On several occasions she fainted and was found to have low potassium levels. Her family urged her to go to the hospital again, but Enid adamantly refused, insisting that she would not submit to treatment that would force her to gain weight. By the time she was 20 she convinced herself that she needed treatment and arranged to come to our hospital after learning that we would not start her on a high caloric diet, but rather would tailor the meal plan to her physiological needs. The meal plan began with 1,200 calories daily and increased in increments of 200 or 300 calories gradually. Despite her willingness to come into the hospital, Enid began to have disputes with the nursing staff from the beginning about the size of her meals and the types of food served. Enid was adept at hiding food from her tray and sequestering it in her room. She would wipe her buttered toast on a napkin, and hide other particles of food that she would later discard. Her bathroom needed to be locked to prevent her from vomiting after meals. Often she would not finish her meals and would attempt to manipulate the staff by giving the nurses and dietitians conflicting information.

During her hospitalization I saw Enid in individual psychotherapy. Her parents, in another state, were not involved because Enid was no longer living at home and had emancipated herself. She wished to separate herself from her parents and had decided to undertake treatment herself. The psychotherapy focused on a realistic discussion of her nutritional needs, on her image of herself, and on her aspirations in life.

Enid had many ambitions and she gradually learned that she could not achieve these while being preoccupied with her obsession to be thin. Her illness had diverted her from her real goals. Despite developing intellectual insight about these issues, she had great difficulty letting go of her obsession to be thin. She saw the anorexia as an ogre who had an unyielding hold on her. She took correspondence courses while in the hospital, keeping up her college studies. Enid slowly gained five pounds, but would lose two or three pounds from time to time and was unable to maintain her weight gain for long. During one month she gained eight pounds and began looking reasonably well nourished. She was able to make her own food choices and maintained this weight for several weeks. We allowed her to return home on a trial basis for two weeks. She had lost four pounds when she returned, but was able to regain this weight in short order. She left the hospital after six months, having managed to gauge her food intake satisfactorily. Within two months her eating habits had again deteriorated and Enid was alternately starving herself and binge eating. She had again started to vomit and she was abusing large quantities of laxatives.

Within the year, she returned and was hospitalized again. Despite her illness she had completed college and maintained an outstanding grade point average. She was somewhat more cooperative in the hospital than at her earlier admission and seemed to make a genuine effort to improve her nutrition. She was adamant, however, about not wanting to weigh more than 95 pounds, which was far from adequate, considering her weight as an adolescent had been 130 pounds. Her main goal was to stop vomiting, and she accomplished this while she was in the hospital. After four more months in the hospital she was discharged to outpatient treatment that continued for another year. Her weight slowly climbed to 103 pounds, as she dealt with issues of her anger toward her parents, her self-esteem, and perfectionism. Enid had made a marginal recovery. Her illness had lasted more than five years, and she was not fully recovered. When she told me that her menstrual periods returned when she weighed 97 pounds, I was skeptical about whether that could be so. However, several years later she was married and became pregnant.

Enid had developed serious complications of her anorexia nervosa. She had to have extensive reconstructive dental work, having her teeth capped because of erosion of her dental enamel from vomiting. She had been rushed to an emergency room on one occasion when she became acutely ill because of a very low potassium level. She was found to have an irregularity of her heartbeat attributable to the low potassium level. As she matured, Enid was able to be less controlled by her disease, but she needed to continue to think about her food intake and structure her meals so as not to starve herself. She eventually married and was able to have two healthy children. Nonetheless, she continued to be scarred by her illness and may never be free from some of its disturbing thoughts.

Because there is such variation among patients, with a wide spectrum of severity, the same treatment does not fit all. Diverse treatments have been used and may be effective in different cases. In my training I was taught that anorexia nervosa is always a serious disease that requires intensive psychiatric treatment. Subsequent experience proved that axiom wrong. Our community study revealed that some individuals recover spontaneously from significant weight loss and from their fear of fatness. Since they did not receive formal treatment we do not know precisely what accounted for their recovery. We say that the recovery was spontaneous because we don't know what happened to incur the positive change toward health. There may have been a nonmedical intervention that resulted in the change. They may simply have become hungry enough to start eating normally again. Their innate biological drive for nourishment may have taken over. They may have consciously realized that they were injuring their health and consequently changed their eating habits. Alternatively they may have responded to the admonitions of their parents or of well-meaning friends. Those who fail to recover by themselves are the ones who tenaciously persist in their desire to remain excessively thin. They are the ones who require treatment and become patients.

If all patients were alike, and if they responded similarly, treatment of anorexia nervosa would be a simple matter. A foolproof formula could be devised that would fit all and assure recovery. Since there is so much variability among patients and among their family circumstances, treatment must be tailored to fit each individual patient's uniqueness. This requires experience, good judgment, skill, flexibility, and ingenuity of the therapist. Inflexible treatment protocols and rigid programs that treat all patients alike should be viewed with suspicion.

In spite of the differences among patients there are some general principles of treatment that are applicable to all. They are to be modified and adapted to the characteristics of the particular patient. The setting of treatment will vary depending on the needs of the patient. Specific techniques are applied to carry out the treatment principles. Finally, the characteristics of the therapist are paramount in determining an effective working relationship with the patient. Let's look at each of these elements.

The Principles of Treatment

Once the person with anorexia nervosa has been evaluated, the diagnosis made, and a measure of rapport established, treatment begins. Some treatment principles can be generalized. The way these principles are applied, however, is a highly individual matter, using various techniques of treatment. There are five principles of treatment that apply to all patients with anorexia nervosa.

Treatment Alliance

The first, and perhaps most important, of these principles is to establish a treatment alliance. The patient must be given the opportunity to develop trust in the therapist. Moreover, the patient and therapist must work toward the common goal to get well. Developing a trusting and working relationship may be difficult to do, but it is necessary for successful treatment. Forming a treatment alliance means working cooperatively rather than having an adversarial relationship. The therapist must demonstrate, by being honest and explicit, that he has the patient's best interest in mind. He may say to the patient, "You and I may not agree on how to get there, but we both have the same goal—for you to get well. I'll listen to you and try to understand what is special about you and how you are different from others, but I know a great deal about your illness and what it takes to get over it. I'll explain the reasons for what we do in treatment and will not deceive you. I hope that I will be able to gain your trust so that we can work together and not against each other."

When choosing a therapist, obviously you want to be certain of his knowledge base: What has been his experience in treating anorexic patients before? Respect and consideration must be evident. Ask yourself if you are comfortable with this physician. Does he answer your questions without being demeaning or condescending?

Weight Restoration

To recover from anorexia nervosa the patient must overcome the effects of starvation and must mature physically. For those in the adolescent years this means undergoing the changes of puberty and catching up with the development that was delayed. Normal puberty is a process that takes several years. Therefore, recovery will take time.

An essential aim of treatment is to restore normal weight. Health cannot be attained while a patient remains undernourished. Thus, adequate nutrition leading to weight restoration is a prerequisite to recovery. Weight gain, however, is not a goal in itself. Too often this has been the focus and measure of success in treatment. Changes in attitudes and behavior must accompany the weight gain if a healthy weight is to be maintained. It is easy enough to restore weight in a hospital with nasogastric feedings or with behavioral treatment, but unless the increased weight is accepted and the distorted perceptions about weight, body shape, and size are altered, the weight that was gained can quickly be lost again. Weight restoration to a healthy weight requires time and patience. The process should not be hastened, especially when undernourishment has been of long standing. The undernourished person has adapted to this state and too rapid re-feeding can be harmful. Obviously, before one can begin to gain weight, one must stop losing it. This requires taking in more food and exercising less in order to counterbalance energy expenditure. The aim is then to increase weight gradually to a healthy level. In a growing adolescent this means restoration of the weight that has been lost, and continued weight gain commensurate with age and developmental level. In an adult, whose growth has been completed, it means restoration of weight to a healthy level. The technique of accomplishing this varies from patient to patient.

Among the youngest patients, who are balking at eating and have not lost much weight, this may mean removing some of the environmental pressures by having the parents stop nagging about eating. Patience and avoidance of conflict at mealtime may allow the child's natural hunger to take over. With many adolescents and adults, outpatient treatment and nutritional counseling are indicated. This is the preferred method leading to weight gain, and it requires gaining the cooperation of the patient. What is involved will be discussed later. The most difficult to treat patients—those in whom the disease has become chronic and those who are steadfastly resistant to changing their eating habits—may need hospitalization where their food intake and weight can be closely monitored. The resultant improved nutrition allows more rational thinking to occur that will, in turn, help to lead to healthier eating habits.

Restoration of Healthy Eating Habits

A more fundamental aim than weight restoration is the normalization of eating habits. This is done through education about nutritional needs. When the illness has been of brief duration, faulty habits may be eliminated without great difficulty. When the habits are firmly entrenched, however, the process will be long and arduous. Younger patients, those who are prepubescent or in their early teens, will often give up their food restriction after a period of treatment. It is as if their natural hunger drive took over, allowing them to eat normally again. Many patients of this age do not need dietary instruction but their parents may need guidance about what kinds of foods to provide. With older teens a dietitian can effectively be involved, as will be described. Initially, the emphasis is on providing adequate calories and later in the treatment a greater variety of food is introduced. Once the patient has overcome her unrealistic fears she can be enlisted to cooperate in striving to become healthy. Older patients and those who have had the illness for a long time require a lengthy period of re-education and nutritional guidance by the dietitian.

Dealing with Emotional Issues

The emotional impediments that have interfered with the patient's well-being are dealt with in psychotherapy with the aim of improving her self-image. Her coping mechanisms need to be strengthened so that she can deal with social pressures more effectively. However, intensive psychotherapy cannot be done while the patient is seriously undernourished. The nutritional state needs to be improved first while empathic support is provided.

The emotional issues that have played a role in initiating and perpetuating the disorder include both elements that anorexic patients share with one another and those that are unique to each individual. Among the shared elements are feelings of ineffectiveness, poor self-confidence, and low self-esteem. Many anorexic patients feel incapable of controlling their lives and consequently strive to control their eating. Moreover, most anorexic patients have distorted views of their bodies and how they see themselves. Additionally, each person with anorexia nervosa has her unique temperament, and comes with experiences that are her own. These general and unique issues are dealt with in psychotherapy. The issues are explored and discussed, and the patient is helped to resolve those that contribute to her illness or are interfering with her life. Often anorexic patients are unaware of their feelings and are incapable of expressing them openly or appropriately. Psychotherapy helps them to recognize and express those emotions.

Working with the Family

Family situations vary greatly. The way that parents should become involved in the treatment depends on the circumstances. The younger the child, the more closely the therapist will want to involve you in the treatment. With adolescents, the intensity with which you are involved in treatment depends on how you are dealing with your daughter's illness and the ways you interact with her. If a great many conflicts have developed in the relationship you may need to be closely involved in the treatment, either by having counseling around those issues or by being involved in family therapy. Adult patients living on their own are usually treated independently of their parents.

As a parent you may feel guilty about being responsible for you daughter's illness. A wise therapist will assure you that you did not cause your child's illness. As was seen in the chapter on etiology, a number of factors interact to bring it about. In order to understand your daughter's aberrant behaviors you must first become educated about the illness. Therapy will then help you to interact with your daughter in ways that enhance, rather than impede, her progress.

The fields of psychiatry and psychology have progressed from blaming parents for most mental and emotional illnesses to a much more sensible recognition that causes of these illnesses are multifactorial. This is emphasized in Harold Koplewitz's book entitled *It's Nobody's Fault.*[1] A more constructive approach than placing blame is to work cooperatively with parents to understand a child's problems and to deal with them effectively.

Parents, however, should not become therapists. An article in the *New York Times* June 11, 2002, discussed a treatment that gives parents the primary responsibility for an anorexic child's recovery. Parents are encouraged to become the therapists and "exhorted to be unwavering in finding ways to feed their child."[2] Often this is exactly what parents have tried to do while their anorexic child becomes increasingly firm in her determination not to eat. Whereas parents' taking control over their child's eating may succeed for some preadolescent children, it could be disastrous for adolescents who have a severe form of the disease. Such an approach really dismisses the therapist's role and places unrealistic expectations on the parents. For treatment to be effective, the patient ultimately becomes responsible for her own recovery. Food issues should be matters of concern between the therapist and the patient, while parents should be helped to disengage from battles about eating. One of the worst scenarios I remember involved parents who were made to understand that they must make their teenage daughter eat no matter how difficult it was. They held her down on the floor and attempted to force feed her with a spoon. Needless to say, this approach failed miserably and totally alienated the daughter from her parents, making her treatment much more difficult. Another "treatment" recommended to be inflicted by the parents was, incredibly, described in a scientific journal.[3] In this aversive behavioral treatment the anorexic patient would receive five painful lashes with a wooden switch whenever she vomited her food or had a "temper tantrum!" Such abominations make a travesty of humane treatment and constitute child abuse. Equally damaging, although more subtle in its harm, is an approach that makes parents feel responsible for causing their child's illness.

Setting the Stage

Melanie, who had become quite emaciated for several years because she drastically restricted her eating, sat looking at her bare arms one morning. For the first time in years she saw herself accurately as she rotated her arms to view them from all angles. She made the startling recognition that her slender bones were barely covered with flesh. This revelation suddenly made her aware that what she had been doing to herself was irrational and it prompted her to seek treatment.

A teenage boy, who had carried dieting to extreme lengths, because of his concern about becoming fat, walked into a shopping mall and saw that people were staring at him. Not until then had he realized that he had become excessively thin, and this realization led him to give up his dieting.

Such sudden awakenings may open the door to effective treatment. The time may come, sooner or later in the course of the illness, when a person recognizes that her control over eating has led to serious consequences and she knows she must change her way of living. Such a realization can begin the process of recovery. Sometimes it leads the person herself to reverse the anorexic process through her own efforts; at other times it guides her to the acceptance of professional treatment. On the other hand, the anorexic person can be stubborn and resistant to the notion of treatment. Engaging that person in treatment can be difficult and time-consuming, and it can require a great deal of ingenuity.

The expectation with which the patient comes to treatment also influences the circumstances under which treatment is begun. I have seen patients who had been ill for years who came to the Mayo Clinic with the high expectation that they would be cured. That expectation gave them the motivation to participate willingly in treatment. Their expectation may be based on factual information, as in the case of Enid. She had read an old edition of the *Mayo Clinic Diet Manual,* in which the gradually increasing diet plan devised by Doctor Berkman for the treatment of anorexia nervosa made sense to her. For others, the expectation to get well and faith in the treatment can become therapeutic forces. Becoming ready to accept treatment is a decisive step in the process of recovery.

Effective treatment requires that the therapist will get to know your daughter who has anorexia nervosa. It requires learning what is unique about her, and understanding her fears as well as her values and aspirations. That is done by listening and by discussing the important issues in her life. This process will take time. There are no shortcuts for bypassing the preliminary work that establishes a trusting relationship. Hilde Bruch believed that the experience of being listened to was of utmost importance in the therapeutic process.[4] It helps to convey genuine interest in the patient. Moreover, it makes the therapist aware of the patient's thoughts and her uniqueness.

Among young adolescents with recent onset of the disorder, the recommendation for treatment from a professional authority, with the parents' support, may carry enough weight to allow her to start treatment, albeit reluctantly. Nonetheless, the therapist will have to earn her trust by being straightforward and honest. Engaging an older person in treatment, one who has been ill for several years after the disease has become a way of life, is more difficult unless something has happened to motivate her. Some such examples were noted above. A motivating factor can be a physical complication that has brought home to the person the seriousness of her illness.

Some patients, often the ones who have been chronically ill, refuse totally to accept treatment. They may seem oblivious to their emaciated condition and to the medical complications it has caused. Every effort should be expended by the therapist to enlist their cooperation through education and sincere persuasion. Rarely, legal constraints, nasogastric tube feeding, or intravenous feeding may be necessary to save a patient's life. However, legal commitment to enforce treatment rarely benefits patients. I have personally never resorted to it. It creates an adversarial stance and often only increases patients' resistance to treatment. They may feel that they must fight the system to preserve their personal integrity. However, I have often firmly told patients that they must enter a hospital to be treated effectively. With parental assent this can usually be accomplished without legal sanctions.

Hospital Treatment

Treatment in the hospital, or inpatient treatment, was in the past often preferred as the treatment of choice because it could provide a comprehensive treatment setting for the patient in a protected environment. It was once falsely assumed that remaining at home was deleterious. But there are other reasons for treatment in a hospital. Although patients almost invariably objected to being in a hospital, they often felt a sense of relief that decisions about eating and exercise would be made for them. The control, which they cherished so much, would be taken from them, but this would ease their emotional burden. Decision making often becomes difficult, even immobilizing, for anorexic patients, increasing their anxiety. Thus, having the hospital staff take charge can reduce this anxiety, although most patients continue to rebel against any external controls.

More often today patients receive outpatient treatment. Most patients can, in fact, be treated effectively as outpatients, but for some this is not enough. While outpatient treatment has the advantages of maintaining the patient in her own environment, allowing her to continue regular school attendance, and giving her the opportunity of making necessary changes in her lifestyle, success is not always possible with this course. Hospital treatment becomes necessary when outpatient treatment is not succeeding, when there is very rapid weight loss, or when medical complications make it unsafe to allow the patient to remain at home. When an associated depression is so severe the patient might attempt suicide, the protection of a hospital clearly is needed. Similarly, when the patient's thinking or behavior is so irrational as to be dangerous to herself, admission to a hospital becomes necessary. In some families where tensions have become high, your doctor may suggest interrupting the conflicts by bringing your teen into the hospital for a time. Finally, hospital treatment becomes necessary when there is no way to provide outpatient treatment within a reasonable distance of the home.

When inpatient or hospital treatment becomes necessary, it should be in a coordinated, well-established program geared to each patient's special needs. There is a place for brief hospitalization on a pediatric unit when a patient is severely dehydrated or has acute electrolyte derangements, but that is only a stop-gap measure to improve the patient's physical state. The underlying illness and the patient's desire to remain thin has not been addressed. Effective hospital treatment takes a long time and is best carried out in a psychiatric unit for adolescents. I am much opposed to mixing children and young adolescents with adult patients on an eating disorders unit. Meeting the developmental needs of adolescence, including a school program, are foremost priorities. Young patients should be with others of their age where suitable activities can be provided. It is more appropriate for adolescents to be with other adolescents, even though they have a variety of emotional disturbances, than to be with adults with eating disorders. Dr. Strober at UCLA emphasizes the value of treating anorexic teenagers in a psychotherapeutic milieu that is congenial and stimulating to their particular developmental tasks.[5]

The establishment of an effective treatment program in a hospital requires a large staff of knowledgeable, devoted professionals and considerable resources. I used to get frequent telephone calls from administrators or nurses charged with setting up a hospital unit for the treatment of eating disorders. Their naïve hope was that I could advise them by phone, or send them a few pages of instructions on how to do it. The sober truth is that it takes numerous well-trained professionals in psychiatry, psychology, nursing, dietetics, and education. Ideally such a program provides comprehensive treatment in a setting that includes a school program. One is most likely to find such a unit at a university medical center or in a large teaching hospital. Unfortunately, limitations in insurance reimbursement have forced some programs to close.

Arnold Andersen, professor of psychiatry at the University of Iowa, has written an excellent description for the clinician of how a hospital program is structured and how treatment in a hospital is delivered.[6] With the diversity of programs now in existence in hospitals and in private residential treatment facilities, it is impossible to list those that are to be recommended on the basis of their quality. A few programs have been models of excellence, however, and have survived for many years. Foremost among these are the programs established by Katherine Halmi at New York Hospital Cornell Medical Center, Westchester Division, White Plains, New York, and that directed by Michael Strober at the University of California at Los Angeles Neuropsychiatric Institute. Your best guide for a recommendation is your physician who is familiar with resources in your region. You can get additional help in finding a program from one of the associations dealing with eating disorders listed at the end of this book.

Realistic goals for inpatient treatment include the restoration of body weight to a healthy level, development of near-normal eating behavior, and attainment of social competence. Clearly, such changes will take time. Sometimes the patient does not maintain them after leaving the hospital, and a second or even third period of hospitalization may be required. Repeated cycles of drastic weight loss and weight gain often lead to chronicity of the disease. This is why it is unwise to shorten the period of hospitalization and to use weight as the sole criterion for hospital discharge. Unfortunately, insurance providers take a short-sighted view. Parents may need to find an advocate—in the treating physician, through an advocacy group, or through legal advice—to help assure that hospitalization will be as long as necessary.

In my view, inpatient treatment encompasses three phases. The first phase involves nutritional rehabilitation when weight loss is stopped, nutritional status improves, and weight gain begins. During this phase the hospital staff takes control over the patient's eating behavior, providing the necessary food portions and setting the expectation that everything is to be eaten. While this aspect of the patient's life needs to be managed by the hospital staff, it is important that her autonomy be respected in other areas so that she does not feel oppressed and hopeless. A balance is to be achieved between controlling harmful behaviors and allowing the patient freedom in other areas of her life. The expectation is for gradual weight gain while the remaining aspects of the patient's life are left in her control. Excessive activity may need to be curtailed, but it is best not to restrict it altogether. The bathroom may need to be locked if she is suspected of vomiting. Emotional support is important during this phase of treatment. This is provided by listening to her concerns, empathizing about her discomfort, but also by pointing out her illogical thoughts and notions. She is required to eat her meals but is assured that she will not be made to become fat. At this point psychological issues concerning family and interpersonal matters are not yet addressed because in the severely starved state, patients are cognitively incapable of dealing with these issues. Throughout this phase the therapist begins to develop a trusting relationship with the patient.

During the second phase, weight comes back into the normal range for adolescent growth while meals are still monitored. At this time the patient is given a bit more autonomy. She is allowed an increased amount of physical activity, taking into account her food intake. Frequent psychotherapy sessions tailored to the patient's individual needs are provided in the second phase. These may deal with interpersonal and family issues, body-image concerns, and self-acceptance.

Finally, in the third phase there is consolidation of the nutritional gains with the patient making her own meal choices and eating more spontaneously. She begins to view herself more realistically and to learn techniques for coping with her family and social surroundings. Psychotherapy continues with emphasis on the patient's future—planning for her return to regular school and reintegrating her into her social sphere. Throughout the hospitalization the family participates in the treatment. The parents are seen by the therapist or social worker with focus on the particular issues that exist. Opportunity for greater independence and autonomy occurs in the third phase as the patient's socialization improves and her sense of humor returns. She may experiment with harmless, mischievous acting out as her adolescent playfulness returns.

Duration of treatment in a hospital varies greatly and cannot be specified except on an individual basis. An arbitrary time period, sometimes dictated by an insurance provider, or the achievement of a specific target weight make no sense regarding a patient's readiness to leave the hospital. Rather, changes that would assure continued progress as an outpatient should have occurred. Foremost among these is the patient's having achieved sufficient comfort around eating for her to be in control of her own eating and maintaining a safe, healthy body weight. The concerns that required hospitalization, such as severe depression and medical complications, should have resolved. A satisfactory level of independent functioning should have been achieved. Exceptionally, a brief period of hospitalization of a few weeks on a pediatric unit may be enough to give successful treatment a start. This requires the availability of good outpatient follow-up. More often, when hospitalization has become necessary, the illness is so deeply ingrained that it takes many months to reverse the pathological process. The inpatient program that we designed at Mayo Clinic in the 1970s and 1980s had a usual length of stay of three to five months. Sometimes, however, a stay of upward of a year or more was required.[7]

Partial Hospitalization

Some programs have turned to partial hospitalization or day treatment as an alternative to hospital treatment, either as a cost-saving expedient or as the preferred method. As in outpatient treatment, the parents are required to be included in the treatment process. Day treatment may be a transition from an inpatient program, or it may be the primary treatment. The program described by Kaplan and Olmsted at the Toronto Hospital is geared to an average stay of 10 to 11 weeks; but like inpatient treatment, to have lasting effects, it often needs to be much longer.[8] Many aspects of treatment, including supervised meals, frequent psychotherapy, and activities with other patients, can be carried out in this setting. Nutritional re-education is a part of the treatment program. Ideally, all three meals should be served in the hospital. Thus the patient can gain a healthier outlook on food and eating.

These treatment programs have begun to fill a need as length of hospitalization has been curtailed and hospital units have been closed. They may be used as a transition from the hospital program to shorten the hospital stay. Because the patient goes home each evening, more personal responsibility is placed on her than if she were in a hospital around the clock, yet she has much more supervision in this program than she would as an outpatient.

Outpatient Treatment

In outpatient treatment the patient remains at home and comes to regular appointments for treatment. In contrast to hospital programs, outpatient status requires active participation by the patient from the outset. She will need to make decisions about her eating based on the recommendations that have been made. This places considerable responsibility on her and makes compliance harder for her initially. However, the changes in her eating behavior tend to be more lasting because the ultimate decisions are left in her hands. An outpatient needs to deal with the environmental pressures that are challenging to her. If she is able to master these pressures and manage her eating in an increasingly healthy way, her capacity to cope effectively will be strengthened. It is easier for the patient to be in treatment in a hospital where she is protected from family stresses and social pressures, but at some point she must return home. This transition can be quite difficult unless her coping mechanisms have been thoroughly strengthened and tested.

For successful oupatient treatment, a patient should start early in the course of her illness before distorted eating habits and other self-destructive behaviors have become firmly entrenched. Old habits are difficult to change. The magnitude of weight loss also has a bearing on the suitability of an outpatient program. Most patients having lost no more than 25 percent of their body weight generally can be treated as outpatients. When 30 percent or more of body weight has been lost, hospital treatment most likely is necessary. Hospitalization is also generally required when the weight loss is very rapid, even though more modest in magnitude. It is difficult to reverse a rapid precipitous loss of weight without hospital support.

A patient's frequency of visits, once her outpatient treatment is established, is usually once a week. Initially she may need to come more frequently to begin establishing a relationship and to have her physical condition monitored closely. When she has made sufficient progress, the therapist may cut her visits to once every two or more weeks. This is dictated by how independently the patient is able to function.

The duration of outpatient treatment may be a few months or several years. It should continue until the patient can manage her nutritional needs independently, has developed a realistic view of herself, and has resumed age-appropriate socialization and activities.

Patient Attributes

Both the patient and the illness itself have characteristics that make treatment easier or more difficult. Most often the person with anorexia nervosa wants to be left alone and forcefully resists change. However, there are almost always positive attributes that support treatment efforts. Almost invariably anorexic patients want to be healthy and strive to improve themselves. It is rare to find one who doesn't want to grow up. Reinforcing the positive aspects of a patient's thinking will promote an alliance with her and enable her and the therapist to work toward similar goals.

Several factors can help treatment efforts:

1. Little weight loss
2. Brief duration of illness

3. Absence of vomiting
4. Absence of binge eating
5. Recognition of thinness
6. Lack of serious emotional disturbance
7. No major environmental hindrances
8. Good family support

Conversely there are attributes that hinder treatment:

1. Great weight loss
2. Long duration of illness
3. Vomiting
4. Binge eating
5. Denial of or unawareness of thinness
6. Serious emotional disturbance
7. Significant environmental contributors
8. Lack of family support

Generally the hindering attributes strengthen the patient's resistance to treatment and reinforce the pursuit of thinness. A patient's tendency to be tenacious and persevering can work either to the advantage or disadvantage of treatment. Used to maintain the status quo, these personality traits are destructive. Redirected, once the patient's cooperation is enlisted, they can be used to work toward positive goals.

What to Look for in a Therapist

Few studies have examined what makes one therapist more effective than another in treating patients with anorexia nervosa. Clearly there are some who do better than others, and differences among therapists can figure importantly in influencing the outcome of the illness. Obviously the therapist must have the inclination and interest to work with anorexic patients. Some shy away from treating these patients because they think it is too difficult or even hopeless.

The therapist should have empathy for the patient and should try to understand the patient's point of view. Conveying the notion of *working with* the patient is of great importance rather than imposing a treatment on her. The therapist you select must be knowledgeable about the illness in order to be competent and to have credibility. He or she must be confident without being dogmatic. There is need to remain flexible as long as it is not detrimental to the patient. Honesty and frankness are other attributes that the therapist should possess because anorexic patients are quick to sense insincerity and deception. Moreover, I believe that patients should be fully informed about their illness, treatment, and progress. Working with anorexic patients requires patience and perseverance. A sense of humor is desirable, especially with adolescents. A long-term commitment to the patient is necessary. Changes in therapists are likely to be detrimental. Even vacations of the therapist are difficult for patients after they have come to rely on him or her. Once a patient has developed a bond with the therapist it is very difficult for her to transfer her trust to another. Every effort should be made for the patient to remain with the same therapist unless the relationship has been unsatisfactory. However, changes should not be made lightly. Just because a patient says that she does not like the therapist should not be reason to make an immediate change. It may be her way of trying to avoid treatment altogether.

The question often arises as to whether one or more professionals should provide the treatment. During my years of practice, I preferred to provide outpatient treatment either by myself or with a dietitian who worked closely with me. Others divide the treatment between a physician, who monitors the patient's physical status, and a therapist—usually a psychiatrist or psychologist—who deals with the emotional and interpersonal issues. Sometimes yet another professional, who may be a social worker, meets with the parents to provide counseling to them. I believe the fewer the professionals involved, the more efficiently treatment can be carried out. Problems of communication among the professionals are minimized and a consistent approach is easier to maintain. When more than one professional is involved in the treatment, it is essential that each has a defined role and that they share the same overall goals for treatment. In day treatment settings, residential treatment programs, and in hospitals, variously constituted treatment "teams" are organized. When they are well directed and coordinated these professionals can function effectively in treating individual patients. When poorly coordinated, however, communication problems are likely to occur, and the patient may pit one professional against another.

Most patients do not need a whole array of treatment modalities, including individual psychotherapy, group psychotherapy, family counseling, support groups, and others. I believe that more is not better, but that these treatments should be used selectively if there are specific indications for them. Knowing when another specialist is needed is the responsibility of the major therapist and is another indication of the importance of establishing an individual relationship with one therapist.

The Role of the Dietitian

A dietitian experienced in the treatment of patients with eating disorders meets with the patient at regular intervals, usually beginning once a week. The chief goal of dietary treatment is to help the patient re-establish normal eating patterns. This can occur after the stage has been set and the patient is willing to make an effort to change her eating habits. With outpatients, this requires at least minimal motivation and a semblance of trust in the dietitian's recommendations. The dietitian must be able to identify the patient's readiness to accept recommendations and to provide fair but challenging goals. These are described to the patient and formulated with the patient if possible.

The dietitian initially obtains a diet history to determine what changes had occurred in the patient's eating habits and to ascertain the current quantity and quality of the diet. Quantity refers to the amount eaten and is usually expressed as the number of calories consumed per day. Quality involves the composition of the diet to assure that it contains a variety of nourishing foods.

A general misconception is that patients with anorexia nervosa have similar dietary patterns characterized by carbohydrate avoidance. In fact, there is much variability in what they eat. Many eliminate fats and starches; others eat an inadequate vegetarian diet. Some eat sweets and little else. Others eat a balanced diet but drastically limit the amounts. Many eat irregularly and go from binge eating to fasting. The aim of dietary treatment is to establish regular meals of good quality and adequate quantity. Diane Huse and I studied 96 patients with anorexia nervosa to determine their dietary patterns. We found that 25 of them ate high-quality meals regularly but simply restricted their calories. Eleven maintained a high quality diet but ate at irregular intervals. Six of these had episodes of binge eating and vomiting or fasting. Sixty patients ate qualitatively poor diets. Among these, 19 consumed regular meals and 41 ate irregularly. Thirty-one of those with qualitatively poor diets were binge eating, fasting, or vomiting, and 30 had idiosyncratic diets. Thus, while all restricted calories resulting in weight loss, there was great variability in how they did this.[9] With such variety, the dietitian must evaluate each patient's diet before determining what changes are to be made. Those who are eating qualitatively poor diets are the most challenging.

The initial diet history forms the basis for the dietary management. A meal plan is designed that considers the current caloric intake as well as food preferences, dislikes, and aversions. Long-standing food dislikes should be distinguished from aversions that have resulted from the disease. With outpatients it is possible to be quite flexible in designing a meal plan, considering the patient's preferences but assuring adequate nutritional composition of the diet. This requires some motivation by the patient and her commitment to do her best to eat the necessary amount of food. Preferably the patient will eat the same foods the family does rather than having to shop for special foods. Low-calorie foods are to be avoided as their use reinforces the dieting pattern. Some allowances can be made, such as using low-fat milk and avoiding visible fats on meat, as long as the overall meal plan is sufficient. A hospital geared to treating patients with eating disorders can't be as flexible as an outpatient program. Otherwise, every patient might want a very different diet. Even so, allowance can be made for particular food dislikes. In our hospital program we permitted each patient three specific dislikes. This worked well in most instances if a dislike was fried eggs, cottage cheese, or pork chops, for example. However, one patient announced that her dislikes were fats, proteins, and carbohydrates. Needless to say, her wishes were unacceptable. Anorexic patients sometimes request a vegetarian diet. This should not be permitted if her interest in vegetarianism was a result of her illness.

When a patient first presents with anorexia nervosa and is ready to make changes to eat more healthily, our first recommendations are aimed at stopping the weight loss. When the weight is stabilized, a meal plan is gradually undertaken that allows weight to increase. We take into account the amount of food that the patient has been consuming. This is estimated by reviewing her diet history. The initial caloric requirement is determined using basal calories, the amount of energy required at rest. This is determined from height, weight, and age. To this must be added the calories needed for activity. In undernourished patients the basal metabolic rate, which is the measure of resting energy requirement (RER), is usually quite low. Therefore, they need fewer calories to maintain their weight than do people of the same weight who are not undernourished. RER can be measured by determining oxygen consumption at rest. Often this is 15 percent or 20 percent below normal. Measuring the RER will predict the caloric content of the meal plan necessary to maintain weight. An amount is added for normal activity and a small increment is added for weight gain. For practical purposes, measuring the RER is often unnecessary and a realistic estimate of caloric need can be made based on the patient's age, height, and weight. The Boothby Berkson nomogram depicted in the *Mayo Clinic Diet Manual* can be used conveniently to determine the initial dietary need.[10] The nomogram is a chart used to estimate caloric requirements based on a person's weight, height, gender, and activity level. The meal plan should be designed first to stop the weight loss or at least to slow it down. It is often in the range of 1,200 or 1,300 calories per day. Patients who have drastically reduced their food intake may need to start with even fewer calories. They may not immediately be able to eat large enough amounts to allow them to gain weight. Within a short time, however, they will need to make an effort to increase their intake, no matter how uncomfortable it is. A meal plan includes foods from each of the basic food groups, with portions enlarged as caloric requirements increase. To begin to gain the trust and confidence of the patient, the dietitian must describe how the initial and ongoing calorie levels are determined. Patients will learn that with weight gain, the signs of semistarvation will diminish. They will experience improved concentration and less cold intolerance and gastrointestinal discomfort such as fullness. These changes increase trust and the focus on wellness, not on weight gain or getting "fat." By discussing the effects of semistarvation, patients usually become more comfortable with the broader needs of their bodies rather than being preoccupied only with weight gain.

Supplementary vitamins are rarely necessary since vitamin deficiencies are infrequent and the meal plan contains sufficient vitamins. The meal plan includes a variety of foods from each food group with the chief deficit being calories. As calories are consistently increased, the nutrient density of the diet increases. While weight rehabilitation occurs with improved food intake, the goal is for individuals to make food choices that result in an adequate diet. A chief concern with adding supplemental vitamins is that individuals usually believe taking vitamins will improve their health and nutritional state regardless of the caloric intake. This mistaken notion is discussed during nutrition therapy.

For patients who have a documented dislike for milk prior to the onset of the eating disorder, a calcium supplement is recommended. Education about and exposure to milk and other dietary calcium sources is an initial goal in nutrition therapy.

With outpatients it is usually desirable for the patient to maintain a food record listing each meal and the quantity of all the foods eaten. This serves as a reminder to follow the meal plan and helps the dietitian monitor progress from week to week. In the hospital, calorie counts are made. Three meals a day are recommended. Snacks may be added depending on the patient's preference and her ability to consume the necessary quantities at meals.

As the treatment progresses, 200 to 300 calories per week can be added. Any excessive activity needs to be curtailed so the patient can gain weight. Weight gain of a pound or two a week is desirable, but this cannot be rigidly enforced. As the patient becomes more comfortable with increased quantities of food, new foods, including those that have been anxiety provoking, are introduced. Anxiety-provoking foods vary greatly among individuals. However, patients often avoid mixed dishes such as casseroles because they are uncertain of the ingredients. Others avoid calorie-containing beverages like juice and milk and prefer to drink diet soda and water. Visible fats, butter, salad dressing, sour cream, sauces, gravy, and cream cheese often cause anxiety because of their fat content. Similarly desserts such as cookies and ice cream are avoided. Sweets including hard candy, jelly, and syrup are less difficult for many to eat.

A goal weight may be set, based on the patient's pre-illness weight or weight percentile. Finally, a maintenance diet is designed to maintain that weight or to induce continued growth in an adolescent who has not reached physical maturity. Throughout the process the patient is encouraged to eat more spontaneously and freely as her fears diminish. Some patients need the guidelines of a meal plan for a long time. Others regain their recognition of hunger and are able to manage on their own.

Diane Huse and I described the dietary aspects of treatment for anorexia nervosa in more detail in the *Journal of the American Dietetic Association*[11] and in the *Mayo Clinic Diet Manual*.[12]

Sample Meal Plans

Two sample menus illustrate the initial and subsequent meal plans for a young adolescent girl with anorexia nervosa. The 1,200 calorie plan represents the initial one for a 13½-year-old girl, 61 inches tall and weighing 70 pounds, who has been eating very little before the beginning of treatment. This may be all that she can tolerate at first. The 2200 calorie plan illustrates her nutritional needs nine months later when she is 63 inches tall and weighs 100 pounds; 50 percent above basal requirement is added for usual activity. Sports or dance participation would require more calories. Older teenagers weighing more will require a greater number of calories to maintain or to gain weight. The dietitian designs a meal plan using food exchanges including adequate amounts in each of the groups: meats, fat, milk, starch, vegetables, fruits, desserts, and sweets. This is calculated to assure an adequate proportion of protein, fat, and carbohydrate. A food exchange list includes foods within each group that contain about the same nutrients. A slice of bread, for example, can be exchanged for one-half cup of cooked cereal in the starch group. Given the meal plan, with a certain number of exchanges the patient can vary her daily menu by substituting foods equivalent in nutritional value.

1,200 CALORIE PLAN
BREAKFAST
1½ cup wheat flakes
2 tablespoons raisins
1 cup skim milk

LUNCH
sandwich: 2 ounces sliced ham
    ½ teaspoon mayonnaise
    1 slice bread
¾ ounce pretzels
carrot sticks
small apple
½ cup skim milk

EVENING MEAL
2 ounces chicken breast
⅓ cup rice
salad: lettuce, tomatoes
    ½ tablespoon salad dressing
    1 cup croutons
1 banana
½ cup skim milk

2,200 CALORIE PLAN

BREAKFAST
1 ½ cup wheat flakes
½ banana
1 cup skim milk
½ English muffin
1 teaspoon margarine

SNACK
Granola bar or
8 snack crackers

LUNCH
Sandwich: 1 ounce cheese
    1 ounce sliced turkey
    1 teaspoon mayonnaise
    2 slices bread
    lettuce
¾ ounces pretzels

1 cup flavored nonfat yogurt
¼ cup dried fruit

SNACK
2 cookies (2 inches diameter)

EVENING MEAL
2 ounces grilled pork chop
1 medium baked potato
2 tablespoons sour cream
1 dinner roll
1 teaspoon margarine
cooked broccoli; 1 teaspoon margarine
½ cup peaches
¼ cup cottage cheese

SNACK
1 small apple
2 teaspoons peanut butter

The Role of Psychotherapy

Psychotherapy is what transpires when the therapist sits down in an office with the patient. During the process of evaluation the two have begun to know each other, and that interaction continues as they meet for regular appointments. A working relationship must first be established. Anorexic patients are typically mistrustful of what will happen to them and they fear that they will be made to gain weight. They may be reluctant to express their concerns because they are emotionally constricted. They may feel that what they say may be used against them or revealed to their parents or to others. Your therapist will likely assure you that what you say is confidential. If you have thoughts of self-harm, that information will need to be shared with the family, but you will be informed that they will be told. By conveying sincere interest in you and by being willing to listen to you, the therapist tries to understand your point of view. It is essential to work together cooperatively rather than antagonistically. As noted above, the experience of being listened to has therapeutic value in itself. It leads to establishment of the bond between patient and therapist. Confidentiality between patient and therapist is important but it should not be carried to extremes by excluding the parents from treatment. The therapist will want to include the parents of a teenager in the treatment to keep them informed about the illness and treatment goals and to enlist their aid in appropriately supporting the patient.

Just as patients differ one from another so do therapists differ in their personalities, styles of relating, and treatment orientations. There is no single best way to do psychotherapy. Thus, a variety of approaches can be effective if they are a good fit for the patient.

Early in the process of psychotherapy a considerable amount of time is devoted to educating the patient about what has happened physiologically during the process of undernourishment. The therapist helps the patient to understand how others see her and how her condition is harmful to herself. Because the patient is usually an unwilling participant at first, it is of utmost importance for the therapist to be forthright and honest. Relatives and others often want to compliment a patient on her looks and initially praise her for her weight loss. This plays in to her delusion that thin is beautiful. It is better to be truthful and to point out the reality that she looks almost like a skeleton. Hilde Bruch said that it is better for a patient to know the painful truth than to be deceived or misled in an attempt to soften the truth.[13] Thus it is the task of the therapist to point out illogical thinking and false perceptions. The patient may be told that she and the therapist may not agree about aspects of her treatment, but they are working toward the same goal—for her to get well.

Therapists once believed that for a patient to understand the emotional conflicts that led to anorexia nervosa would be therapeutic in itself. However, focusing on these issues alone may help her understand her psyche, but it does not change her eating behavior. Once the physical changes associated with starvation are well under way, they take on a life of their own and are not easily reversed. Some anorexic patients are adept at discussing emotional issues from the past in an intellectual way while avoiding their real feelings. Through psychotherapy these patients can be helped to recognize their emotions in order to deal with them more realistically. Psychotherapy should address the patient's current functioning and her maladaptive behavior, and provide techniques to help her cope and adapt.

In my training I was once advised to avoid the topics of food and eating with my anorexic patients and rather to deal with the "real underlying issues." Inevitably, though, these topics came up, so I have learned to use them because of the patients' remarkable interest in nutrition. This logically leads to discussing their growth and development and the physiology of starvation and weight gain. In my experience it makes sense to let patients know what they weigh and how their weight changes from week to week. Some therapists hide this from their patients. This serves no purpose other than deceiving the patient. It does not really allay their fear of gaining weight. It is better for them to know the facts than to leave them guessing. If they want to know their weight they can easily weigh themselves elsewhere. With many patients I made use of growth charts and weekly graphs of weight to review their progress and to discuss adolescent growth and development. Once they accepted the goal of getting well they often responded to encouragement and praise. Various devices can be used to motivate the patient and to increase her pride in her accomplishments. For example, you may reward some patients by letting them participate in sports after they have made a certain amount of progress.

When she is severely undernourished, the patient cannot deal with many psychological issues because her ability to think logically has failed. As her nutritional state improves her capacity to think logically improves as well. Psychotherapy can then explore the patient's family interactions and other interpersonal relationships. The direction such discussions will go depends on the individual issues and concerns that are important to the patient. Efforts are made to understand the patient's life at present and her thoughts about herself, her family, her friends, and school. The patient's regrets and reasons for impaired self-esteem are also explored. These discussions will solidify the therapist's understanding of the patient and continue to strengthen his or her relationship with her.

Before long, the therapist needs to address the patient's aspirations and goals for the future. In working with adolescents, in particular, he or she should emphasize the future rather than the past. As mentioned earlier, a sense of humor is desirable in the therapist. Working with adolescents requires spontaneity and innovation. While it is necessary to emphasize the seriousness of the illness, the tone of treatment should be light and optimistic when possible.

A variety of techniques are used in psychotherapy to enhance the patient's ability to express herself. Patients who are not readily verbal can benefit from the use of art as a therapeutic technique. Some can use written stories and poetry to express their feelings. These can help the therapist understand the patient's unique concerns and can lead to discussion of issues that the patient otherwise could not express.

Much has been written about the techniques of psychotherapy with anorexic patients. This evolved largely from the work of Hilde Bruch. She explicitly described how she talked with her anorexic patients in *The Golden Cage* and *Conversations with Anorexics*.[14,15] She used techniques similar to what is now known as cognitive-behavioral therapy. David Garner, Kelly Vitousek, and Kathleen Pike have described this technique in great detail in the *Handbook of Treatment of Eating Disorders*.[16] With any treatment, the wisdom of the therapist comes into play. Applying someone's technique indiscriminately will not work. Thus, techniques of treatment must be adapted to the needs of each individual patient.

The Role of Medication

Because anorexia nervosa is an illness that is highly complex and often difficult to treat, some therapists have used medications to try to enhance weight gain and to shorten the course of the illness. Unfortunately there is no medication that is specific for the treatment of anorexia nervosa. Over the years a wide array of medications has been tried including hormones, vitamins and minerals, appetite stimulants, and psychiatric medications. None has proven effective either in curing the illness or in shortening its course. Some therapists have tried to alter the physiological changes that result from starvation. This does not affect the underlying disease mechanism. At one time patients were given thyroid extract to increase their metabolic rate because it is low in anorexia nervosa. However, the patient's caloric requirement would thus be increased as well. Unless she ate considerably more, she could experience even greater weight loss, and the treatment would be hazardous. Appetite stimulants are not warranted because the problem in anorexia nervosa is not lack of appetite but unwillingness to eat.

Sufficient sources of calcium—milk and milk products—need to be included in the diet to help build bone during adolescence and to prevent osteoporosis. Vitamin and mineral supplements are not a substitute for food. They have no value in themselves; they are needed to metabolize the foods eaten. Thus, an adequate balanced meal plan will contain the necessary vitamins that are naturally present in a variety of foods. Even so, your doctor may want your teen to take a daily vitamin and calcium supplement to assure that she is getting these elements. But taking them should not be seen as a substitute for any foods and should not be a reason to eliminate certain foods from the meal plan.

Sometimes psychiatric medications are used to augment the treatment of patients with anorexia nervosa. However, anorexic patients are inherently suspicious of medications because they fear these will make them gain weight against their will or exert control over them. They usually resist taking medications. Nonetheless, there are situations when medications may appropriately be used as part of the treatment. When patients have profound symptoms of depression, anxiety, or obsessive thinking, certain medications, particularly the selective serotonin reuptake inhibitors (Prozac, Paxil, Zoloft and others) may be helpful. Because an undernourished person is more prone to side effects, a smaller dose than usual is indicated. Patients need to be educated about the reasons for a particular medication's use, and their cooperation must be gained if it is included in their treatment. Remember that patients in general very often will not take prescribed medications. They may refuse or forget or just consider taking it to be inconvenient. The cost of the medication may also be a deterrent, but this is relatively small compared to the other costs of treatment.

When binge-eating and vomiting are present, certain medications have been used to reduce the urge to eat excessively. Tricyclic antidepressants (desipramine and imipramine) were once used but are now largely avoided because of their side effects. The selective serotonin reuptake inhibitors (particularly Prozac and Zoloft) have been found effective to reduce bingeing and vomiting in the short term but their effect is often not lasting.

Anorexic patients usually don't need medications during the early phases of treatment when their nutrition is impaired. Sometimes medications are used to reduce the anxiety they experience with eating. Later in the course of treatment, however, once their nutrition has improved, depressive symptoms may persist or supervene for some. These are manifested by listlessness, poor concentration, difficulty in making decisions, feelings of worthlessness, and social withdrawal. Antidepressant medications, particularly the selective serotonin reuptake inhibitors, may then have a place in the treatment. By this point a trusting relationship with the therapist has been established and the patient is more likely to agree to the medication if the therapist carefully explains the reasons for taking it.

In summary, there is no medication that specifically treats anorexia nervosa, but medications may be helpful in alleviating certain symptoms associated with the disorder.

CHAPTER THIRTEEN

Is Recovery Possible?

Patients often keep diaries or write stories and poetry that express their feelings about their experiences. These can provide sharp insights into their illness that they have difficulty expressing otherwise. Such writings can be used effectively in their treatment, and they also can provide some insights into the recovery process.

Two years after she first came for treatment, I asked Frances to write her recollections of her illness. In retrospect, she had some vivid recollections of her thoughts and feelings. She had been unable to describe these feelings at the time she was undernourished. When she was first undergoing treatment she denied that anything was wrong. Here is some of what Frances wrote about her illness and her recovery.

Suffering from anorexia was the most suffocating, horrible pain I have ever felt. I became so self-absorbed I could think of nothing else, except what I looked like and what I weighed, what others thought of me, and how much I'd eaten that day. I can remember counting over and over in my head the number of fat grams and calories I had eaten that day, and always purposely overestimating so I was sure that I wasn't eating more than I thought I should. I became an expert on the amount of fat and calories in every single food. At school, after lunch, the number of calories I had eaten would consume my thoughts for the rest of the day, so much that I really don't know how I got through the rest of the afternoon, let alone my senior year, with nearly straight A's, when I was the sickest.

At that point in my life, I was very unhappy. I had absolutely no self-esteem. I internalized everything, causing me to distance myself from family and friends, and I cried myself to sleep many nights. I would not only cry because of the physical pain of lying on a protruding hipbone, but I also cried thinking to myself, "I just want to be normal." I didn't see how everyone else my age could be so happy in their imperfect bodies when I was so miserable, but however they did it, I envied their confidence and happiness. I knew the unhappiness that I was feeling wasn't normal, but I honestly didn't know what was wrong with me.

Another big problem that I faced was being really compulsive with exercising. If I ran five miles one day, the next day I would have to run six, and then the next day even more. Or, if I rode an exercise bike for forty minutes one day, the next day I would think that I had to top that. I would exercise until absolute exhaustion. I had no energy to keep going, but I had more willpower than at any other time in my life, so frequently I kept it up until nearly passing out.

As a physical repercussion of the disease, my skin was constantly dry and chapped. My hands and feet turned a yellowish-orange color and my hair became really thin and brittle. I also stopped menstruating for almost two-and-a-half years. People often told me that I looked gaunt and lifeless.

Denial was another big part of my anorexia. Although people commented daily that I was too thin or sick, or asked me what was wrong, I never saw myself as thin. I denied everything and wondered how everyone else could be so wrong and blind. Although I knew I was losing weight, since I weighed myself several times each day, I still never thought I was thin enough. I always had the thought that, "If only I could be thinner, then I would be happy and have a perfect life." Every time the scale showed a reduction in my weight, I felt powerful and as though I had more control of my life. Likewise, I felt powerful when I would deny myself food. Others gave in to and indulged in food.

Even as I ordered children's sized pants, and as doctors administered test after test, several even reacting accusingly as though I was doing this to myself on purpose, even as I was forever cold and uncomfortable as I sat in a chair or car, I still saw much more fat that I thought I needed to get rid of.

Getting fat was an intense fear of mine. I remember several times nearly hyperventilating, when I didn't know what I would eat in a certain situation, or when the only food available was in my mind too fatty. My throat literally felt like it was closing up and tears would well up in my eyes as I sat there paralyzed by fear. I became very unsociable, because I didn't want to have to deal with any food situations where I would be uncomfortable, and I often refused to eat in front of other people.

I am not sure if my lack of self-confidence was a result of the eating disorder, or vice versa. Whichever it was, I had so little confidence in myself that I couldn't even bring myself to go out for the basketball team anymore, had I been healthy enough to play, even though I have always loved the sport. I also quit other activities that I had previously been involved with and most of the time tried to avoid people.

I had certain hours that I could and could not give myself permission to eat. For example, breakfast was always the same—a banana and a bagel—and I absolutely did not eat again until after noon. Then I could only allow myself to eat a very small snack before dinner if I was really hungry, but I was happiest if I didn't need to resort to that. I refused to eat dinner until at least six-thirty and I always ate very slowly, taking very small bites.

Unfortunately, it took forceful efforts from my parents and friends to get me to accept professional help, because I truly didn't think that I was eating disordered. I didn't think it could be possible to be happier if I gained weight. Even after I began treatment, it was a long time until I recognized that I needed help and even longer until I actually wanted to get better and gain weight. The first time I ever remember wondering if I looked OK, as far as gaining weight is concerned, was my senior year at the prom, which was a while after I had started improving physically. I remember thinking that I hoped I didn't look gross (meaning too thin) and that I looked OK, a huge improvement for me.

However, once I did get help, I was happier and more full of life than I ever remember being before, and it was the best thing I ever did. I gained so much confidence and self-esteem that had been missing in my life for so long and it was a great relief and almost a "ReLife!" I finally realized and accepted that I am much more than just a physical body and am worthy enough to allow myself to be taken care of.

What Frances wrote of her experience typifies the thoughts and actions of many others who had anorexia nervosa. Most are quite unable to express their thoughts and feelings at the time of their illness, and few can describe them so poignantly after they recover. At the time of her illness she denied much of what she became able to recognize later.

Bonnie was 70 years of age when I spoke with her about her reminiscences of her illness. She was a small, tanned, sinewy, lean woman with a weather-beaten face; she exuded energy. Retired from a career as a medical secretary, she was now volunteering in a nursing home. All but one of her four grown children were residing nearby and she was very much involved with them and her grandchildren. She had been treated by Doctor Berkman back in the late 1940s. He first saw her when she was 19 years of age. The previous winter, shortly after Word War II had ended, she had begun to diet. Over a year's time her weight fell from 150 pounds to 106. At the time of the examination in the following autumn she weighed only 76 pounds fully dressed. She described feeling distended after eating and wondered whether she had an intestinal obstruction. The examination revealed cold intolerance, dry skin, and fear of obesity. Doctor Berkman's plan was to start her at the Diet Kitchen (a cafeteria supervised by a dietitian where special dietary needs could be met) with a meal plan amounting to 1,300 calories daily. That was gradually increased to 3,200 calories. In addition, he prescribed a sedative to reduce her anxiety and overactivity. The food quantity was gradually increased every few days. Doctor Berkman continued to see her during the subsequent years. Her weight reached 88 pounds when she was 22, but again fell to 74 pounds a year later. Doctor Berkman noted briefly in the medical record, "This has been an up and down affair." By age 27 she weighed 106 pounds. He considered her nearly recovered. He would have liked to see her reach 120 pounds for a year or two. She married and became pregnant soon thereafter, even before her menstrual periods had resumed. Her first child was born when she was 28. Two other children followed in quick succession, and a fourth child when she was 35.

Bonnie was eager to talk about her illness and how she remembered it. She had never kept it hidden and had often volunteered to talk to teenagers who were struggling with the disorder, or to a parent who was overwhelmed by her daughter's dieting. Regarding her own experience, she mused, "I've often wondered if you ever really, really, recover, or if it's like an addiction where you're always something like a recovering alcoholic. There's that awful fear of getting fat."

"You had mentioned to me that you still have the thought that if you gained a lot of weight you'd still get upset about it," I replied.

"Yes, I wonder if I would start to take those diet pills or something like that again."

"What would make you gain a lot of weight, do you think?"

"I don't know—the only thing I'm thinking is because of where I work. People are in wheelchairs and are so sedentary, they don't move, and some of them just explode out because all they're doing all day long is eating. It takes them an hour to eat and then they get wheeled back to their room. They're in their bed, they come out, and they eat again."

"Are you still keeping active physically—do you exercise?"

"Oh, yes. I go Monday, Wednesday, and Friday to the Health Club and I lift weights for about half an hour and then I do aerobics for an hour. This is the seniors class—so you have to be at least 50, and I think I'm the oldest. In the summer I'm still biking and I do my walking. When this gal and I were timing ourselves we got down to 11½ minutes per mile, but its probably more like 15 to 17 minutes now. And it depends on who you're walking with."

"Do you worry what would happen if you couldn't exercise?"

"I wouldn't like it. It probably would frustrate me, but I wouldn't panic. I'm an active person. I'm not into sitting and knitting."

"Do you watch what you eat now?"

"I don't think I pay attention to it, but I've gotten in a habit of eating vegetables and fruit and oatmeal and bran and stuff, and that's pretty much what I stick to. I haven't had meat for years, but I have cheese now and then."

"Do you know how many calories you consume?"

"Not any more—I'm sure I knew every calorie I ate for a while."

"Do you get the necessary calcium?"

"Yes, because greens usually have calcium—your broccoli and . . . "

"Do you drink milk?"

"I don't like dairy foods so much. Just if I put it on cereal."

"Is it skim?"

"Yes, that's all we have in the house. My doctor wanted me to go on estrogen and I refused that, but I said that I would start taking Tums to get the calcium. I'm not one that goes to the doctor often—about every 10 years or so. I've had three bike accidents which caused me to go to the hospital. Years ago I had two broken ribs. The doctor said this was happening for lack of calcium. I was just sitting in a car and we hit a bump and when I came down two bottom ribs cracked."

"Did you ever have a test for bone density?"

"Yeah, and I guess that went OK."

"Now let me ask how it all began."

"I remember when the dieting began. And the reason I remember it was one of the first paychecks we got, which was 75 bucks a month. So we had a party. It was my first experience drinking. I don't know where the gals got the booze from because none of them were old enough. I was 19. I always weighed in the 140s in my high school days. But I was solid as a rock, about 5' 3" or 4". We had a party and I ended up getting extremely sick. I spent my money on chips because we never had booze in the house. The gals whose parents had booze in the house got something from the booze cupboard, and none of us knew how to drink, and we were all sicker than dogs. So that was on a Friday. I didn't go back to work until Tuesday because I was so sick, and I know there was polio season around, and mother thought I might be coming down with that. I had reached 150 pounds and when I went back to work I was back down to 142. So I had lost 8 pounds, I think. I don't know that I ever ate breakfast. Then I'd have a grapefruit and an apple for lunch. And supper, I don't know—I just picked away at what we had. And, of course, I got all kinds of kudos from family and friends. I don't think I wanted to be real thin and I wasn't into the stylish figures. But I think I was heavier than the gals I ran around with, and I wanted to get down to their weight. But it wasn't on my mind a whole lot. Just the opportunity was there to lose some weight. I think my mother spotted it before I went out to California. She said it was getting a little ridiculous. But when I was out there I was kind of having a ball being in charge.

"That was near Hollywood and I worked for this doctor. He wanted me to replace his nurse. I would take patients in the room and get them ready for the exam. So then I was basically on my own. I weighed 112 when I left for California. I was 68 when I came back."

"And nobody noticed it out there in California?"

"He never mentioned anything about my weight."

"But it must have been obvious to people."

"You know who it was obvious to—college students. There was a big fruit stand a couple of blocks from where I lived. I'd go out there every night and stock up on fruit and these students who took medical courses would ask 'What else do you eat besides this fruit?' They noticed that I'd lost weight. And at noon I'd go to this little drug store and get buttermilk and another college student came and sat beside me and said, 'You know, I think you got a disease.' And I said, 'No.' He said, 'Three months ago you had more weight on you.' But I always felt good, and so I never—you don't look at the mirror—you look at the scale.

"I always felt good so I had no concerns, just had tons of energy. And I'd stopped menstruating and that didn't bother me because I started so late anyway. I didn't know that should be something to be concerned about. There were two nurses who rented another room who thought that something was really wrong with me and they started giving me Vitamin B shots. But then they said I should see a doctor. And he just said that they're concerned that I had cancer. So after he examined me he said, 'No, you couldn't have cancer, I'd feel any lumps that you had.' So he said I was probably homesick and I should go back home. So when I got home—my mother worked in a clinic. So I went in there and walked in and she was working with a patient and I waited. She said 'You'll have to wait outside until your name is called.' Three times she sent me out, and it dawned on me she doesn't really recognize me. So when she came out again I said, 'Mom!' And she said, 'Oooh!'

"Poor thing. I think of that quite often. I was expecting this big, 'Hello, I'm so glad you're home.' She kind of tried to keep from crying and said, 'Let me finish up here.' I think she probably called Dad to give him a warning.

"They never really preached at me, which I think helped, and they probably knew I was very independent. Then Doctor Berkman talked to my Dad about the Diet Kitchen. When I got back home they used to have these roaming photographers on the street and they'd put your picture on a postcard. They took a picture of me, and I was shocked to death. I could *not* believe that that was me. The wind was blowing and my skirt was blowing between my legs and my knobby knees were— oh, it was just—it really got me thinking. That's when I consented to go to the Diet Kitchen.

"Tell me how you first met Doctor Berkman—what he was like."

"He was really nice. I never got the sense that he was preaching to me or that I had done something wrong. He just kind of asked a lot of questions—he was very curious. How things got started and how long I'd been at it, you know, and if I was feeling OK. They did a barium swallow and stuff, to see if things were passing through my system, and to make sure if there wasn't another medical problem. If I would start getting upset about things then I would call him and he would say, 'Well, come on in and talk to me.'

"I try to remember over at the Diet Kitchen, because you always cheated when you first went in. It was a big shock. It looked like enough food for eight people. A few things would go into my pocket—like my dessert—or I'd take something home. I can't down it now, but I'll take it home and I'll eat it, but of course I never did.

"Then there was a gal that was getting different food from what I was getting. She was trying to spice up things—not such a heavy meal, instead of all the gravy and butter and stuff. I noticed that type of food went through better.

"What was the treatment like?"

"It was mainly the Diet Kitchen. I could quit there when—I think they wanted me at 92 pounds, and that was a struggle. And then I think, at 82 I just refused to go and mainly because I knew it was costing Dad a heck of a lot of money. And I said I could do it on my own. I did get up to 92. I would stick at the 2's—72, 82, 92—and you know, for months I couldn't break that, and once I'd break that and get up to 102."

"You said that Doctor Berkman never blamed you, or said it was your fault. Did you feel that it was your fault?"

"No, not a real fault. I just felt guilty for what I put Mom and Dad through, and yet maybe not guilty enough. I still wanted to control that part of it. I went through a real religious time there, too, like I'd feel guilty if I made a mistake on the typewriter. I was at church praying every morning. And this all went along with the guilt I was feeling— disrupting the family. But I don't know that anybody ever blamed me. I got the guilt from something, but not like you're a bad girl. You're just crazy to do that to yourself."

"You felt badly that you were doing this to your family, but did it ever occur to you that your health was being harmed?"

"Never. Maybe if I'd gotten sick. I would have reacted differently, but, no,—never, really."

"Did you think about your body much at all—about how you looked?"

"I don't think so, as I say, I never looked in the mirror. But I knew if I put on a few pounds that would bother me. I'd always put it on my stomach and would feel it there. If it had only gone on my arms or something, where I wanted it. But I wasn't into the models that are held up as a goal for people. I was too much into the activities and sports and stuff. Whatever was available to girls those days."

"To what do you attribute your recovery? What do you think made you well?"

"I think probably getting married had something to do with it, and then I got pregnant so fast. They didn't think I'd be able to have children because it was so long since I had had a period."

"You got pregnant before you had a period, didn't you?"

"Yes. In fact, I did have a spotting. I remember calling Doctor Berkman. He said, 'Now don't get excited, just come in and get examined.' Well, I was pregnant then. We'd been married four months. So I think in that taking on—all of a sudden I had other people to worry about and take care of. I was planning meals, and I had never thought of food before. I was 98 before I got married and then I got up to 109 and stayed there for many years, I gained 45 pounds with the pregnancy and then I got down to 109 and stayed there."

Bonnie made a successful recovery from anorexia nervosa. She was able to stabilize her weight at a physiologically safe but slender level. She led a productive, satisfying life. She regained her fertility and bore four healthy children. Once she had achieved her normal weight, her austere diet and lifelong exercising may, in fact, have had health benefits in preventing obesity, heart disease, diabetes, and high blood pressure. Her mind is still very active and interested in new things at age 70. Nonetheless she has vestiges of distorted thinking about weight. She is at risk of osteoporosis and fractures, although she has not had a serious fracture. She will probably outlive many of her contemporaries.

Long ago when the parents of a teenager with anorexia nervosa would ask me, "What is your success rate in treating this disease?" I would answer, "It depends," because I knew the outcome depended on many factors. I did not know, in fact, what would happen some 10, 20, or 30 years later to the many patients I had treated. I knew what had become of them one or two years after their treatment, but I also knew that was not nearly long enough to tell the whole story. I also knew that the outcome depended on many factors other than my skill in treating the disease. Some of these had to do with the severity of the illness, innate characteristics of the patient, and circumstances that would exacerbate or ameliorate the disease. I knew that none of my patients had died, that many of them were getting better, but that some were continuing to struggle with their disorder.

Outcome, in fact, varies tremendously. Some young women make a full recovery; unfortunately, a few may die of the illness. We do not have good predictors of eventual outcome so that at the onset of the illness it is not possible to be sure who will recover and who will not.

Betty was 20 years of age when she came to medical attention because of a 25-pound weight loss during the previous year. She weighed only 99 pounds. Despite her weight loss she was active and said that she had a good appetite. No obvious reasons for the weight loss were found on her examination and laboratory tests. After she graduated from high school she had become obsessed about her weight and tried unsuccessfully to lose some pounds. When her childhood sweetheart broke up with her she believed it was because she was fat and she renewed her efforts to diet. This resulted in marked weight loss, and her menstrual periods ceased. When she saw the physician she expressed the belief that she was still fat and insisted that she was eating plenty.

The physician who saw her suspected that Betty was not eating as much as she claimed. He recommended that she eat more and outlined a diet plan sufficient in calories to induce weight gain. A month later she returned, having gained six pounds. She had also become engaged to a young man whom she met at work. Subsequently she married and a year later she had continued to gain weight and became pregnant. She delivered a premature but healthy infant.

Throughout her life Betty was in very good health and weighed around 150 pounds. She never had a recurrence of the weight loss that she experienced in young adulthood. After age 75 she developed osteoporosis and broke her hip. Her memory began to fail; she had a downhill course, and died of Alzheimer's disease when she was 85 years of age.

Betty had a mild form of anorexia nervosa from which she recovered without intensive treatment. Undoubtedly, emotional factors played a role in instigating the problem. Fortunately, her notion of being fat did not persist. The illness resolved before there were serious complications. Her successful marriage and the birth of her child helped her to focus on others rather than on herself. Being accepted by her spouse bolstered her self-confidence. She became less introspective and focused on caring for her child. Thus her need to diet dissipated. It is doubtful that her osteoporosis was related to her relatively brief duration of undernutrition. She evidently recovered in all respects.

In contrast, Rose began to restrict her diet when she was 24 because she thought that her hips and stomach were too chubby. She progressively lost a considerable amount of weight during the next few years and her menses ceased. She was a valued bookkeeper in a retail clothing store, a hard worker; she was full of nervous energy and constantly in motion. She never married and continued to live at home with her elderly parents. Her weight loss progressed to the point that she appeared emaciated, her arms and legs becoming mere sticks. Fine downy hair appeared on her forearms and on her sunken cheeks. Her employer repeatedly urged her to seek medical help but Rose found numerous excuses to avoid this. Finally, she was warned that her employment was in jeopardy unless she had a medical evaluation. The physician diagnosed anorexia nervosa and recommended that Rose enter a hospital for treatment. Rose refused and promised to increase her food consumption. She told her employer that no medical cause for her undernutrition was found and that everything would be fine. She told him, moreover, that as long as she was performing her job, her health was her own business.

Rose continued to perform efficiently at work but gradually seemed to lose even more weight. Over the next few years her complexion grew sallow and her body took on a cadaverous appearance. Nonetheless, she seemed to have abundant energy and she continued to be indispensable and highly productive at her job. She would not disclose her weight to anyone, even her family members. As she neared middle age she began to feel more easily fatigued and no longer displayed the energy of former years. Her family repeatedly urged her to seek medical care, but Rose never pursued this beyond a brief medical evaluation. At age 41, her family brought her to an emergency room because she had fallen asleep that day and had become unresponsive. She was found to be in a state of collapse and moribund. She had a cardiac arrest, was resuscitated, and admitted to the hospital. All attempts were made to keep her alive, but within a few hours her heart stopped again, and she died. Rose simply starved herself to death.

These two cases represent the two extremes in the outcome of anorexia nervosa. Betty recovered fully even without receiving intensive treatment. She lived a long life free of the concerns she once had about her weight. Her case is not unique. Our community study showed that it is not unusual for a teenage girl to have all the hallmarks of anorexia nervosa, yet to recover fully without treatment after some months or a year or two. Rose, in contrast, developed chronic anorexia nervosa over a decade and a half, becoming progressively more undernourished, and eventually died of her disease. Still others have recurrences of their illness punctuated by marked weight fluctuations over the course of years. Some develop a chronic form of the disease and may remain at a borderline level of acceptable weight for much of their lives. Some of these women live a long and active life. A few die of their disease. Depression may be an accompaniment of the disorder, and some take their own lives in their 20s, 30s, or 40s. Not infrequently they begin abusing alcohol, which plays a role in the suicide. Death may occur from electrolyte abnormalities. Among these are persons who have developed bulimia nervosa, characterized by binge eating and vomiting, as a sequel to anorexia nervosa.

When one reviews follow-up studies and studies of outcome in anorexia nervosa, one is confounded by a mass of conflicting information. In some studies, three-quarters or more of the patients recovered; in others, only half recovered from their illness. Individual outcomes vary so greatly that group statistics are of little use in helping us to know how any one individual will fare. Reports of mortality associated with anorexia nervosa are even more confusing. In some studies none had died; in others more than 20 percent of the patients had died at the time of follow-up. There are numerous reasons for these discrepancies. The diagnostic criteria were inconsistent; some studies used broader while others used stricter definitions of the disorder, and patient groups varied in the severity of their illness. The settings from which the patients were selected varied, and the length of follow-up differed markedly. Patients who were in hospital programs are likely to have been more severely ill, while those who received outpatient treatment tended to be less ill. There was variation in the duration of their illness prior to treatment, and treatment methods differed. The longer the duration of follow-up, the greater the likelihood that the patient had died.

In many studies mortality was reported as the crude mortality rate (CMR), simply the percentage of patients who had died of any cause. To arrive at a truer picture of mortality, one should compare the number of observed deaths to the expected number of deaths in the general population. This is expressed as the standardized mortality ratio (SMR).

George Hsu reviewed the world literature regarding outcome of anorexia nervosa and found much variation in reported outcomes.[1] Mortality in different series of patients varied as much as from 0 percent to 19 percent, but in over half the studies reviewed the mortality rate was below 5 percent. There was much variation in weight recovery and in patients' social and emotional functioning.

Clinicians like to attribute changes in behavior to treatment, but they may fail to recognize that many things happen in the life of an individual that affect, alter, and influence their lives and their illnesses. These other influences may have as strong or stronger an impact on an illness than the treatment. Time can heal.

A more practical question than asking what percentage of patients recover is, "How long will the illness last?" Most clinicians treating anorexic patients do not have the opportunity to follow their patients' course for many years. Therefore, the long-term outcome remains generally unknown. The longest follow-up study was done by Sten Theander in Sweden.[2] He found that relapses may occur after several decades, and that recovery can occur even after as long as 12 years. Theander identified 94 females with anorexia nervosa who were treated in general medical and psychiatric clinics of southern Sweden from 1933 to 1960. He reviewed the status of these women at several time intervals and found that 71 patients (76 percent) had ultimately recovered after 24 years or more. However, a disturbing number, 10, had died of anorexia nervosa and 5 by suicide. Two additional patients had died of cancer. Six patients had developed a chronic course of the illness and still had symptoms. This study paints a discouraging picture with a very high mortality rate. This is tempered by the fact that the patients were severely ill and had required hospital treatment. Theander, however, did not compare the number of deaths to the expected mortality rate of nonanorexic women of like age. A reassuring finding of the study was that recovery could occur even after more than 12 years. Most important, the great majority of patients—three out of four—eventually recovered.

Dr. Michael Strober is a psychologist at the University of California in Los Angeles and editor of the *International Journal of Eating Disorders*. He and his colleagues painted a much more optimistic picture.[3] Their study of 95 adolescents with severe anorexia nervosa who were hospitalized at the UCLA Neuropsychiatric Institute provides a more encouraging view of the outcome of anorexia nervosa than appears in other research. The study was a methodologically refined one with careful follow-up. Patients were followed prospectively for up to 15 years from the time of their admission. They received intensive treatment in the hospital, generally for several months, and they continued to have outpatient treatment after discharge from the hospital. The study results revealed that 76 percent achieved full recovery after 10 to 15 years and 86 percent achieved partial recovery. Full recovery was defined as sustained weight recovery and absence of deviant attitudes regarding weight and shape, including worry or rumination over weight, weight gain, or need for control of eating and weight. Partial recovery required the attainment of normal weight and normal cyclical menstruation. Particularly gratifying was the finding that no patients in this group had died. This supports my clinical impression that death from anorexia can usually be prevented with careful treatment and follow-up. Nonetheless, significant weight loss following hospital discharge was common, and recovery often required many years. Some of the patients remained chronically ill. The longer the patients remained ill, the less was the likelihood of recovery. Because the study was published as recently as 1997 and the patients were adolescents at the time of hospitalization, reports on their outcome into middle age and old age must await future follow-up. It is possible, of course, as Theander's study suggested, that some may relapse in the future.

More than 40 years after I first treated patients I still believe that outcome depends on many factors. At the onset of the disorder I do not believe that one can predict what will happen to any one individual. I know from having seen many hundreds of patients and from reviewing the medical charts of hundreds more in our epidemiological study that the outcome is extremely variable. What impressed me most is how patients eventually differed one from another even though they looked remarkably alike at the time of their starvation disease. Many of my former patients have kept in close touch with me, and I have learned about others after several decades. Some of their stories are recorded in this book. Most have recovered from their illness and have become well-functioning, contributing members of society. A good many have become the mothers of healthy children. However, some have remained chronically undernourished and are making only a marginal social adjustment.

At Mayo Clinic we studied everyone in the community of Rochester who had had anorexia nervosa between 1935 and 1989, regardless of whether they received any treatment. This study differed from other follow-up studies in that it included all the persons with anorexia nervosa and was representative of the illness in the community. It painted a vivid picture of the natural history of the illness. Its most striking finding was that the outcome was extremely varied, with most subjects recovering. A few died of anorexia nervosa or of complications related to the illness. In this study we followed 208 patients (193 women and 15 men) for up to 63 years from the onset of their illness. The surprising finding was that the number of deaths was no greater than was expected for Minnesota women and men of similar age in the general population (standardized mortality ratio 0.71). In other words, for the entire group, anorexia nervosa did not increase their risk of dying prematurely. To be sure, eight women and one man died of causes possibly related to their anorexia nervosa at the ages of 27 to 71. Of these, one died of starvation at age 41, two died by suicide at ages 33 and 47, and six died of complications of alcoholism at the ages of 27 to 71. While the great majority of anorexic patients do not die of their illness, our study suggests that there is an increased risk of suicide, and a number of patients develop problems with alcohol, most likely some of those who had become bulimic.[4] While our study makes for a hopeful tone in that most patients can expect to recover, it should not lead to complacency about treatment because some will indeed die of their illness.

The relationship of anorexia nervosa and alcoholism is not well understood. One would think that anorexics would avoid alcoholic beverages because of the calories contained. It is true that most young anorexic patients avoid alcohol not only for this reason but also because drinking is against their value system. Some, however, begin drinking eventually and may become alcohol dependent. The drinking consequently is beyond their conscious control. Some may begin drinking because they are depressed and some are genetically vulnerable because of alcoholism in their families. Alcoholism is known to be overrepresented in families of anorexic patients.

How many individuals die of anorexia nervosa nationwide? The National Center for Health Statistics reported only 145 deaths annually between 1986 and 1990 that were attributed to anorexia nervosa.[5] This is undoubtedly an underestimate because anorexia nervosa is often not noted on death certificates even though the illness contributed to the death. It means, though, even if one increases this number several fold, that there are far fewer deaths than publicized in the media. Extrapolating from our community data and based on the population of the

United States, we can estimate that there are 750 to 1,500 deaths annually attributable to anorexia nervosa. Fortunately, this number is smaller than has generally been estimated. To put this number in perspective, three-quarters of a million persons die each year in the United States of heart disease and a half-million die of cancer. Accidents kill 100,000 people, 69,000 die of diabetes, and 29,000 commit suicide.[6]

These varied and conflicting results confirm that anorexia nervosa is a diverse illness. Many will recover completely from a single episode of anorexia nervosa during adolescence. Others go on to have recurrences of their illness into adulthood, and some remain chronically anorexic without ever becoming well. A few die of their illness, rarely from the effects of starvation itself. A significant number of those who die do so by suicide, as a result of electrolyte derangements, or from alcohol complications. This wide range of outcomes indicates that anorexia nervosa does not have the same implications for each individual. It can be a relatively mild, transient occurrence or it can be a very serious illness even leading to death. For most, it is intermediate in severity, lasting for several years before complete or partial recovery occurs.

CHAPTER FOURTEEN

Can Anorexia Nervosa Be Prevented?

If only we could prevent anorexia nervosa we could avoid the complicated treatment for this tenacious disorder. Undeniably, avoiding it would be better than treating it once it is under way. But whether prevention is possible in those who are the most vulnerable is highly questionable, and educational efforts aimed at prevention may actually increase the occurrence of anorexia nervosa by heightening a youngster's excessive focus on diet, nutrition, and body awareness.

Data on prevention are sparse. School-based preventive programs have been attempted with elementary, middle school, and high school students with the aim of improving their self-esteem and teaching them about good nutrition. These interventions also inform young women and men about the health hazards associated with eating disorders. Most children should benefit from such knowledge and they will if they understand and assimiliate the information in a constructive manner. Those who are already vulnerable to developing anorexia nervosa, however, may ignore the information or it may encourage them to become even more engrossed in unhealthy preoccupations.

The largest study of preventive efforts was conducted by Killen and others at the National Institute of Child Health and Human Development in Bethesda, Maryland.[1] It included data from several areas around the United States. The researchers reported the results of a preventive school curriculum designed to modify the early attitudes and unhealthful weight regulation practices of almost a thousand sixth-

and seventh-grade girls. The program taught healthy weight management and skills to resist societal pressures. Posttesting showed that the girls' knowledge increased but their attitudes and behavior did not change. After completing the study the authors questioned the wisdom of providing a curriculum directed at all young adolescents, most of whom are not at risk to develop an eating disorder. They felt that it might be better to focus on students who are at high risk.

Identifying those students is problematic, however, and exposing them to this education could prove risky because it might even heighten their overconcern about their diets and bodies. Young students are more likely to be influenced by media advertisement and by their peers than by well-intentioned adults.

In another study, Mann and colleagues had college students who had recovered from eating disorders provide information about their experiences to female college freshmen.[2] At follow-up the intervention group actually had more symptoms of eating disorders than did the controls. The authors felt that the stigma of the disorders may have been reduced, and thus, having eating disorder symptoms became more acceptable. Vulnerable girls might identify with these former anorexics and there is the risk of glamorizing the disorder.

Niva Piran, a psychologist who has studied prevention of eating disorders extensively at the University of Toronto, wisely pointed out that preventive programs are likely to fail unless there is intervention with significant adults in the life of the children—parents, teachers, coaches, and physicians.[3] Expecting children and adolescents to change their behaviors without reinforcement in their social environment is unrealistic. More efforts aimed at informing these significant adults is warranted.

Carter and his co-workers attempted a school-based prevention program for young adolescent girls designed to reduce dietary restraint. While there was an increase in their knowledge and a temporary reduction in their dietary restraint, over the long run there was actually an increase in dietary restraint.[4]

Girls most at risk for developing anorexia nervosa are unlikely to use knowledge they gain in preventive curricula in a constructive manner. Many anorexic patients are already very knowledgeable about nutrition. They have memorized the caloric content of most foods, and they are informed about recommendations for healthy eating. The problem is that they have taken the information too seriously and have applied it inappropriately during a time when their bodies are growing and they need plentiful nourishment.

Another pitfall of preventive programs is that they focus on only a few factors that are associated with anorexia nervosa. The widespread messages of the media and of advertising extolling thinness are likely to have a greater effect. The temperamental and personality characteristics that make a girl vulnerable cannot easily be changed. There is speculation that in the future genetic engineering could offer preventive hope by altering a person's vulnerability to the harmful effects of dieting. However, the genes that determine temperament and personality traits likely interact with environmental influences in complex ways. Some of these genes may contribute in positive, as well as negative, ways to the makeup of the individual.

According to Battle and Brownell, researchers working at Yale University, public health measures would likely have the greatest impact on preventing both eating disorders and obesity.[5] Obesity is by far a greater public health problem than is anorexia nervosa. Unfortunately, the measures aimed at preventing obesity, when carried out assiduously, are conducive to development of anorexia nervosa. Reducing the availability of calorie-dense fast foods and snack foods, encouraging the increased consumption of fruits and vegetables in the diet, and increasing physical activity could decrease the incidence of obesity. These are the same measures that potential anorexic patients use. Thus the preventive measures might actually increase the occurrence of anorexia nervosa in vulnerable individuals.

Among the factors that help set the stage for anorexia nervosa in young girls, cultural values that favor thinness have perhaps the greatest impact in our society. These values are ubiquitous in magazines and on television. The fashion industry perpetuates the images of ultra-slim models. Most teen idols are thin. In the 1960s it was Twiggy; in the twenty-first century it is Britney Spears.

The only effective prevention, to my mind, is early individual intervention with those children and young adolescents who begin to show the signs of anorexia nervosa. Those who have become overzealous about dieting and exercise, those who are not gaining weight commensurate with their growth, and those who are not maturing physically. The best hope for prevention is to stem the progression of the illness before it becomes severe. This can be done within a family by providing firm, yet sensitive, nonjudgmental guidance. It can be done by a concerned friend or adviser. It can be done by the affected person herself if she becomes aware of the irrationality of her behavior, and if she becomes informed about the consequences of self-starvation. It can be done by a pediatrician or family physician who can help the person to stem the progression of the illness in its early phases.

As noted above, the school-based prevention programs may do more harm than good, unduly focusing the attention of vulnerable students on their bodies. Effective prevention would require a wholesale change in the priorities and values expressed in our society. Such changes could diminish the cultural pressures to diet. But changing the thrust of marketing and advertising is unlikely to happen. For now the most realistic hope for prevention is to identify those with early symptoms of anorexia nervosa and to provide prompt individualized treatment.

Can death from anorexia nervosa be prevented once the illness has begun? I believe it can. Empathic treatment should be instituted as soon as possible. This requires a therapist forming an alliance with the patient and establishing a long-term relationship until the negative aspects of the illness are overcome. I believe that optimism about outcome is warranted and that most patients will get well.

What Parents Can Do

There is ample evidence that the cultural influences in our society set a high premium on thinness. Superficial beauty is valued above substance. These ubiquitous messages affect even young elementary schoolchildren and have a powerful impact on adolescents. They come to believe that they will be judged by how thin they are and how they compare to their idols—popular singers, models, and actresses. A high-paced lifestyle has changed family life so that children have little supervision over what they eat. Family meals and regular meals have been replaced by hasty meals consumed on the run and by snacking.

How can parents counteract these influences? Most important, parents should communicate with their children and listen to their concerns. Adolescents may become less communicative with their parents, but by being available and patient their parents can stay in touch. Even though adolescents may not agree with their parents they will be aware of their parents' values and priorities. Parents should set an example by valuing positive attributes over superficial appearance. They should provide regular meals and encourage a balanced variety of foods. They should provide education about the need for substantial nourishment during the time of rapid growth during adolescence.

If some warning signs of anorexia nervosa appear, parents can deal with them directly. Persistent food avoidance, particularly of fats and meats, failure to gain weight, and excessive exercise are some of these signs. Parents should frankly express their concerns and discuss the need for appropriate nutrition with their teen. By being alert to changes in eating habits and behavior, parents can avert problems before they become firmly established. Recognizing children's achievements and attributes unrelated to their physical appearance can bolster their self-esteem and self-worth. Children should also be encouraged to show concern for others rather than being overly involved with themselves.

If the problems persist, a meeting with the pediatrician or family physician is indicated; he or she will determine the seriousness of the situation. Identified early enough the problems often can be reversed. Once they are well established, more intensive treatment is needed. Families can play a crucial role in setting positive examples and in teaching children values that are salutary and health promoting.

This book will be read by parents, family, friends, and others including professionals. I want to address a few words especially to you—the patient. I hope that you will read the book too. Anorexia nervosa is a serious illness that can become devastating and ruin your life. But as I showed, it's possible to recover from it. You may not like to be called a patient because you believe that you are well. But you've become a patient once dieting and weight loss are out of control and harming your body, and you've been taken to see a doctor about it. It may be hard to accept that your dieting and striving for perfection has become an illness. In addition to the toll anorexia nervosa takes on your emotions, it causes you to have trouble concentrating and will eventually make you weak and fatigued. As starvation progresses your body will suffer and you will risk harming your heart, kidneys, and brain. All this will keep you from enjoying your life.

By seeing your doctor and getting treatment you will have to do some things that you don't want to do, particularly after you have worked so hard to become thin. You will need to make some changes in your eating habits and perhaps to exercise less. You will need to gain some weight so that your body can regain strength, endurance, grow and develop, and function normally again. The process of treatment will help you to recognize your feelings and to come to grips with the things that have been bothering you. It's not so much about weight, but there may be other things that you don't like about yourself. I hope that this book has given you some insight into how anorexia nervosa develops in different people, how they deal with it, and how each individual differs. It also shows the way it harms you.

I hope that you will see that your doctor and therapist should be you ally and advocate; not your enemy. To overcome anorexia nervosa you will have to do some things that you do not want to do, such as eating more, and eating foods that you have avoided. The process of treatment will be hard and sometimes painful. You will feel like fighting the treatment but I hope that you will be able to trust your doctor and therapist to do what's in your best interest. When you recover and can stop being a patient you will be thankful that you did the necessary things to work cooperatively with them. When things are hardest they will be there for you.

It's up to you.

A number of nonprofit resources in the United States and Canada provide advocacy, information, educational materials, and listings of professionals who provide treatment for people with eating disorders. Some sponsor self-help groups. Such groups bring together individuals and families of individuals with eating disorders. They provide mutual support and disseminate information but are not a substitute for professional treatment.

As yet there is no single organization analogous to the American Cancer Society or the American Heart Association that acts as an advocate for people suffering with eating disorders, but there is movement in that direction. One of the oldest groups, the American Anorexia/ Bulimia Association, based in New York, has merged with the National Anorexic Aid Society to become the National Eating Disorders Association. Some states have separate organizations.

The Academy for Eating Disorders, founded in 1993, is an organization of professionals and lay persons with an interest in eating disorders. Their directory of members can be a helpful guide to locating a qualified professional, but as with any referral list, it is wise to get a personal recommendation from your physician or other trusted person who knows that professional. The websites shown below provide specific information about each group. Some include links to other resources.

AACAP
American Academy of Child and Adolescent Psychiatry
3615 Wisconsin Avenue NW
Washington, DC 20016
Telephone: 202-966-7300
Website: http://www.aacap.org

The professional organization for child and adolescent psychiatrists. In addition to sponsoring professional meetings for scientific exchange among members, the organization provides information for families and advocacy for child mental health. Website provides information on developmental, behavioral, and mental disorders affecting children and teenagers. Facts for Families give information on many issues that affect children, teenagers, and families. Information on when and how to seek help for your child and referral service for finding child and adolescent psychiatrists, psychologists, and social workers.

AED
Academy for Eating Disorders
6728 Old McLean Village Drive
McLean, VA 22101
Telephone: 703-556-9222
Website: http://www.aedweb.org

A multidisciplinary association of professionals advocating in the field of eating disorders. Sponsors an annual conference. Provides a list of members who are active in the treatment of individuals with eating disorders.

Membership requires an advanced degree and training and experience in the field of eating disorders.

Anyone, including lay persons who are interested, may become an affiliate member.

NEDA
National Eating Disorders Association
603 Stewart Street, Suite 803
Seattle, WA 98101
Telephone: 206-382-3587
Tollfree: 800-931-2237
Website: http://www.NationalEatingDisorders.org

Provides advocacy, information, referrals, and support groups.

ANAD
National Association of Anorexia Nervosa and Associated Disorders
P.O. Box 7
Highland Park, IL 60035
Telephone: 847-831-3438
Website: http://www.anad.org
Provides advocacy, information, referrals, and support groups.

ANRED
Anorexia Nervosa and Related Disorders, Inc.
Website: http://www.anred.com
This organization has merged with NEDA but maintains a separate informational website.

The National Eating Disorder Information Centre
CW 1-211, 200 Elizabeth Street
Toronto, M5G 2C4, Canada
Telephone: 416-340-4156
Toll-Free: 866-633-4220
Website: http://www.nedic.ca
Provides information and resources on eating disorders.

U.S. Department of Health and Human Services
The National Women's Health Information Center
8550 Arlington Blvd., Suite 300
Fairfax, VA 22031
Toll Free: 800-994-9662
Website: http://www.4woman.gov
Provides health information including information about eating disorders.

U.S. Department of Health and Human Services
National Health Information Center
P.O. Box 1133
Washington, DC 20013
Toll Free: 800-336-4797
Website: http://www.health.gov/nhic
A health information referral service. Puts health professionals and consumers in touch with organizations that answer health questions.

PREFACE
1. Sullivan, PF, Discrepant results regarding long-term survival of patients with anorexia nervosa? Mayo Clin Proc. 2003; 78:273–274.

CHAPTER ONE
1. Bruch, Hilde, The Golden Cage, The Enigma of Anorexia Nervosa, Cambridge, Mass., Harvard University Press, 1978, p. vii.
2. PBS Television Documentary, "Dying to Be Thin," Dec. 12, 2000.
3. Wolf, Naomi, The Beauty Myth, How Images of Beauty Are Used Against Women, New York, William Morrow, 1991, pp. 179–183. While the statistics she cites grossly overstate the incidence, prevalence, and death rate from anorexia nervosa, Wolf poignantly describes her own self-starvation as an adolescent. Her style of writing is colorful and incisive, if overly dramatic. The paperback version (New York, Anchor Books, 1992) deletes the statement that 150,000 American women die each year of anorexia nervosa, and notes that the number who die is unknown.
4. Center for Disease Control, National Vital Statistics Reports, 2002; 50:1-31.
5. Brumberg, Joan Jacobs, Fasting Girls, The Emergence of Anorexia Nervosa as a Modern Disease, Cambridge, Harvard University Press, 1988. Historian Brumberg is professor in the Department of Human Development and Family Studies at Cornell University. A scholarly historical and sociocultural analysis of anorexia nervosa from the feminist perspective.
6. Tolstoy, Leo, War and Peace, Translated by Louise and Aylmer Maude, The Great Books, University of Chicago, Encyclopedia Britannica, 1952, p. 372. Describes Natásha's illness, which puzzled her doctors when she could not eat or sleep, and grew thin after breaking off her engagement.
7. Bemis, KM. Current approaches to the etiology and treatment of anorexia nervosa, Psychological Bulletin, 1978; 85:593–617.

CHAPTER TWO

1. Gottlieb, Lori, Stick Figure, New York, Simon & Schuster, 2000. A revealing story of a young girl's struggle with anorexia nervosa based on Gottlieb's diaries.

CHAPTER THREE

1. Hsu, LK George, Eating Disorders, New York, Guilford Press, 1990. One of the best concise treatises on eating disorders for the professional and the informed lay person. Hsu has distilled a great deal of research evidence into this highly readable synthesis of current knowledge.

2. American Psychiatric Association, Diagnostic and Statistical Manual of Mental Disorders, fourth edition (DSM-IV), Washington, D.C., American Psychiatric Association, 1994.

3. Theander, S, Anorexia nervosa: a psychiatric investigation of 94 female patients. Acta Psychiatr Scand [Suppl] 1970; 214:1–194. Theander's classic monograph that became the basis for the first long-term follow-up of patients with the disorder. The subjects for study were selected from a region in southwestern Sweden where they had been treated between 1931 and 1960.

4. Innes, G, Sharp, GA, A study of psychiatric patients in North-East Scotland, J Ment Sci 1962; 108:447–456.

5. Kendell, RE, Hall, DJ, Hailey, A, Babigian, HM, The epidemiology of anorexia nervosa, Psychol Med 1973; 3:200–203.

6. Jones, DJ, Fox, MM, Babigian, HM, Hutton, HE, Epidemiology of anorexia nervosa in Monroe County, New York, 1960–1976, Psychosom Med 1980; 42:551–558.

7. Smukler, G, McCance, C, McCrone, L, Hunter, D, Anorexia nervosa: a psychiatric case register study from Aberdeen, Psychol Med 1986; 16:49–58.

8. Willi, J, Grossmann, S, Epidemiology of anorexia nervosa in a defined region of Switzerland, Am J Psychiatry 1983; 140:564–567.

9. Lucas, AR, Beard, CM, O'Fallon, WM, Kurland, LT, Anorexia nervosa in Rochester, Minnesota: a 45-year study, Mayo Clin Proc 1988; 63:433–442. Our community-based study of the incidence and prevalence of anorexia nervosa identifying patients beginning in 1935.

10. Lucas, AR, Beard, CM, O'Fallon, WM, Kurland, LT 50-year trends in the incidence of anorexia nervosa in Rochester, Minn.: a population-based study, Am J Psychiatry, 1991; 148:917–922. An additional five years was studied to bring the study up to 1985.

11. Lucas, AR, Crowson, CS, O'Fallon, WM, Melton, LJ III, The ups and downs of anorexia nervosa, Int J Eat Disord 1999; 26:397–405. Updates the study for an additional five years through 1989, for a total of 55 years.

12. Hoek, HW, Brook, FG, Patterns of care of anorexia nervosa, J Psychiatr Res 1985; 19:155–160.

13. Råstam, M, Gillberg, C, Garton, M, Anorexia nervosa in a Swedish urban region: a population-based study, Brit J Psychiatry 1989; 155:642–646.

14. Crisp, AH, Palmer, RL, Kalucy, RS, How common is anorexia nervosa? A prevalence study, Brit J Psychiatry, 1976; 128:549–554.

15. Soundy, TJ, Lucas, AR, Suman, VJ, Melton, LJ III, Bulimia nervosa in Rochester, Minnesota, from 1980 to 1990, Psychological Medicine 1995; 25:1065–1071. The first study of incidence of bulimia nervosa in a community.

16. Russell, G, Bulimia nervosa: an ominous variant of anorexia nervosa, Psychol Med 1979; 9:429–448. The first description of a new syndrome, which Russell named bulimia nervosa.

17. Russell, GFM, Anorexia nervosa through time, in Szmukler, G, Dare, C, Treasure, J eds., Handbook of Eating Disorders, Chichester, John Wiley, 1995, pp. 3–17.

18. Hoek, H, The incidence and prevalence of anorexia nervosa and bulimia nervosa in primary care, Psychological Medicine 1991; 21:455–460.

CHAPTER FOUR

1. Weiner, Herbert, Psychobiology and Human Disease, New York, Elsevier Publishing Company, 1977.

2. Engel, GL, The need for a new medical model: A challenge for biomedicine, Science 1977; 196:129–136.

3. Lucas, AR, Toward the understanding of anorexia nervosa as a disease entity, Mayo Clin Proc 1981; 56:254–264. Based on the talk "A century of progress," given at a symposium on anorexia nervosa held in Denver in 1978 when Hilde Bruch was awarded the Mt. Arey Hospital Gold Medal for her lifetime achievements in the understanding of eating disorders. In the talk I suggested the biopsychosocial model for the pathophysiology of anorexia nervosa. The paper in the Mayo Clinic Proceedings also defines historical eras in the study and treatment of anorexia nervosa.

4. Hamer, Dean, and Copeland, Peter, Living with Our Genes, New York, Doubleday, 1998. Written for the layperson, this book explores how genetics determines not only susceptibility to physical illnesses but much about personality characteristics.

5. Ibid.

6. Ridley, Matt, Genome, The Autobiography of a Species in 23 Chapters, New York, Harper Collins, 1999. A delightfully written book about how human traits are determined by heredity. An example is given chapter by chapter for each human chromosome.

7. Gelehrter, TD, Collins, FS, Ginsburg, D, Principles of Medical Genetics, second edition, Baltimore, Williams & Wilkins, 1998. An authoritative textbook of medical genetics containing basic principles and clinical applications.

8. Erlenmeyer-Kimling, L, Vulnerability research: a behavior genetics point of view. Yearbook, Internat. Assoc. of Child Psychiatry and Allied Professions, 1978; 4:45–49.

9. Keys, A, Brošek, J, Henschel, A, Mickelson, O, Tayor, HL, The Biology of Human Starvation, Minneapolis, University of Minnesota Press, 1950. The classic work on the effects of starvation based on the study of volunteer conscientious objectors during World War II at the University of Minnesota. It is still the most comprehensive source of information about the physical and psychological effects of starvation.

10. Crisp, Arthur, Anorexia Nervosa, Let Me Be, London, Academic Press, 1980.
11. Hsu, LK George, op. cit.
12. Shandler, Sara, Ophelia Speaks, Adolescent Girls Write About Their Search for Self, New York, Harper Perennial, 1999.
13. Peters, SD, Wyatt, GE, Finkelhor, D, Prevalence, Ch. 1 in Finkelhor, DA, ed., Sourcebook on Child Sexual Abuse, Beverly Hills, Sage Publications, 1986, pp. 15–59.
14. Laporte, L, Guttman, H, Abusive relationships in families of women with borderline personality disorder, anorexia nervosa and a control group, J. Nerv. & Mental Dis 2001; 189:522–31.
15. Pfeiffer, RJ, Lucas, AR, Ilstrup, DM, Effect of anorexia nervosa on linear growth, Clin Pediatrics 1986; 25:7–12.

CHAPTER SIX
1. Academy for Eating Disorders, 6728 Old McLean Village Drive, McLean, VA 22101, (703) 556-9222. Email: aed@degnon.org., Website: http://www.aedweb.org

CHAPTER SEVEN
1. Winokur, G, Munoz, R, Feighner, J, Robins, E, Guze, SB, Woodruff, RA, Diagnostic criteria for use in psychiatric research, Arch Gen Psychiat 1972; 26:57–63.
2. American Psychiatric Association, Diagnostic and Statistical Manual of Mental Disorders, fourth edition (DSM-IV), Washington, D.C., American Psychiatric Association, 1994, pp. 544–545.
3. Garrow, JS, Crisp, AH, Jordan, HA, et al., Pathology of Eating Group Report, in Silverstone, T, ed., Appetite and Food Intake, Berlin, Abakon Verlagsgesellschaft, 1976, pp. 405–426.
4. American Psychiatric Association, Diagnostic and Statistical Manual of Mental Disorders, third edition (DSM-III), Washington, D.C., American Psychiatric Association, 1980.
5. American Psychiatric Association, Diagnostic and Statistical Manual of Mental Disorders, third edition, revised (DSM-III-R), Washington, D.C., American Psychiatric Association, 1987.
6. Frisch, RE, Demographic implications of the biological determinants of female fecundity, Soc Biol 1975; 22:17–22.
7. Frisch, RE, McArthur, JW, Menstrual cycles: fatness as a determinant of minimum weight for height necessary for their maintenance or onset, Science, 1974; 185:949–951.
8. Garrow, JS, Webster J, Quetelet's index (W/H^2) as a measure of fatness, Internat J Obesity, 1985; 9:147–153.
9. Bruch, Hilde, Eating Disorders, Obesity, Anorexia Nervosa, and the Person Within, New York, Basic Books, 1973. Bruch's classic book in which she summarized her early studies in obese children, and her later work on anorexia nervosa.
10. Bruch, H, Perceptual and conceptual disturbances in anorexia nervosa, Psychosom Med 1962; 24:187–194.
11. Frisch, RE, op. cit.

CHAPTER NINE

1. Lucas, AR, Callaway, CW, Anorexia Nervosa and Bulimia, Ch. 238, in Berk, JE, ed., Bockus Gastroenterology, fourth edition, 1985, pp. 4416–4434. Contains a detailed discussion of the physiological and hormonal changes in anorexia nervosa.

2. Abel, TL, Malagelada, J-R, Lucas, AR, Brown, ML, Camilleri, M, Go, VLW, Azpiroz, F, Callaway, CW, Kao, PC, Zinsmeister, AR, Huse, DM, Gastric electromechanical and neurohormonal funtion in anorexia nervosa, Gastroenterology 1987; 93:985–965.

CHAPTER TEN

1. Treasure, JL, Wheeler M, King EA, Gordon PA, Russell GF, Weight gain and reproductive function: ultrasonographic and endocrine features in anorexia nervosa, Clin Endocrinology 1988; 29:607-616.

2. Sobanski E, Hiltmann WD, Blanz B, Klein M, Schmidt MH, Pelvic ultrasound scanning of the ovaries in adolescent anorexic patients at low weight and after weight recovery. European Child & Adolescent Psychiatry 1997; 6:207–211.

3. Lucas, AR, unpublished data.

4. Dr. Elizabeth Mussey practiced obstetrics and gynecology at Mayo Clinic from 1947 until 1974, where she saw many undernourished patients with anorexia nervosa. She had Dr. John Berkman see the difficult ones who needed more than supportive encouragement.

5. Starkey, TA, Lee, R, Menstruation and fertility in anorexia nervosa, Am J Obstetrics and Gynecology 105:374–379, 1969.

6. Russell GF, Treasure J, Eisler I, Mothers with anorexia nervosa who underfeed their children: their recognition and management, Psychological Medicine 1998: 28:93–108.

CHAPTER ELEVEN

1. Russell, G, Bulimia nervosa: an ominous variant of anorexia nervosa, Psychological Medicine 1979; 9:429–448.

2. Soundy, TJ, Lucas, AR, Suman, VJ, Melton, LJ III, Bulimia nervosa in Rochester, Minnesota, from 1980 to 1990, Psychological Medicine 1995; 25:1065–1071.

3. Kendler, SK, MacLean, C, Neale, M, Kessler, R, Heath, A, Eaves, L, The genetic epidemiology of bulimia nervosa, Am J Psychiat 1991; 148:1627–1637.

4. Fairburn, CG, Beglin, SJ. Studies of the epidemiology of bulimia nervosa, Am J Psychiat 1990; 147:401–408.

5. Lucas, AR, "Pigging Out," JAMA 1982; 247:82.

6. Wynn, DR, Martin, MJ, a physical sign of bulimia, Mayo Clinic Proceedings 1984; 59:722.

7. American Psychiatric Association, Diagnostic and Statistical Manual of Mental Disorders, fourth edition (DSM-IV), Washington, D.C., American Psychiatric Association, 1994, pp. 545–550.

8. Ibid., Appendix B, pp. 729–731

CHAPTER TWELVE
1. Koplewitz, Harold, It's Nobody's Fault, New York, Times Books, 1996. A very readable and sensible guide to children's emotional and psychiatric disorders providing reliable information for parents seeking a diagnosis and treatment for their children.
2. New York Times, June 11, 2002. Article reviewing Lock, J, le Grange, D, Agras, W S, Dare, C, Treatment Manual for Anorexia Nervosa: A Family-Based Approach, New York, Guilford Press, 2001. This treatment manual gives explicit guidelines for family treatment with verbatim reports of what transpires in treatment sessions. This approach may be effective for younger adolescents in experienced hands but cannot be generalized to all patients.
3. Blue, R, Use of punishment in treatment of anorexia nervosa, Psychological Reports 1979; 44:743–746.
4. Bruch, H, Anorexia nervosa: therapy and theory, Am J Psychiat 1982; 139:1531–1538.
5. Strober, M, Yager, J, A developmental perspective on the treatment of anorexia nervosa in adolescents, Ch. 16, in Garner, DM, Garfinkel, PE, eds., Handbook of Psychotherapy for Anorexia Nervosa and Bulimia, New York, Guilford Press, 1985, p. 384.
6. Andersen, AE, Bowers, W, Evans, K, Inpatient treatment of anorexia nervosa, Ch. 7, pp.327–353, in Garner and Garfinkel handbook. Earlier, Anderson wrote, Practical Comprehensive Treatment of Anorexia Nervosa and Bulimia when he was at Johns Hopkins University (Andersen, A.E., Practical Comprehensive Treatment of Anorexia Nervosa and Bulimia, Baltimore, Johns Hopkins University Press, 1985) which provides practical guidelines for all aspects of treatment and lists resources available throughout the United States. With changes in personnel over time this list has inevitably become out of date.
7. Lucas, AR, Duncan, JW, Piens, V, The treatment of anorexia nervosa, Am J Psychiat 1976; 133:1034–1038.
8. Kaplan, AS, Olmsted, MP, Partial hospitalization, Ch. 18, in Garner, DM, Garfinkel, PE, eds., Handbook of Treatment for Eating Disorders, second edition, New York, Guilford Press, 1997, pp. 354–360. The Handbook is a comprehensive multi-authored compendium on treatment modalities for professionals. The first edition (Garner, DM, Garfinkel, PE, eds., Handbook of Psychotherapy for Anorexia Nervosa and Bulimia, New York, Guilford Press, 1985) brought together chapters by numerous authorities and became the standard reference volume on treatment.
9. Huse, DM, Lucas, AR, Dietary patterns in anorexia nervosa, Am J of Clinical Nutrition 1984; 40:251–254.
10. Nelson, JK, Moxness, KE, Jensen, MD, Gastineau, CF, Mayo Clinic Diet Manual, seventh edition, St. Louis, Mosby, 1994, pp. 303–311. Successive editions of the diet manual have included sections on the nutritional management of anorexia nervosa. Early editions specified the dietary progression recommended by John Berkman.

11. Huse, DM, Lucas, AR, Dietary treatment of anorexia nervosa, J Am Dietetic Assoc 1983; 83:687–690. Describes principles of treatment, taking the diet history, determination of caloric content of the initial diet, diet progression, and weight gain expectations. An expanded version of this paper including sample meal plans and menus was published as Treatment of anorexia nervosa: dietary considerations, Ch. 21, in Frankle, RT, Dwyer, J., Moragne, L, Owen, A., eds., Dietary Treatment and Prevention of Obesity, London, John Libbey and Co., Ltd., 1985, pp. 201–210.
12. Nelson, JK, Moxness, KE, Jensen, MD, Gastineau, CF, op. cit., pp. 655–666.
13. Bruch., H,. The constructive use of ignorance, in Anthony, EJ, ed., Explorations In Child Psychiatry, New York, Plenum Press, 1975, pp. 247–264.
14. Bruch, Hilde, The Golden Cage, the Enigma of Anorexia Nervosa, Cambridge, Mass., Harvard University Press, 1978. A popular book in which Bruch described case histories illustrating the thoughts of anorexic patients and Bruch's technique of psychotherapy.
15. Bruch, H. Conversations with Anorexics, Czyzewski, D, Suhr, MA, eds., New York, Basic Books, 1988. Published posthumously and edited by Czyzewski and Suhr, this was Bruch's final work based on her dictated manuscript. Bruch had made tape recordings of her psychotherapy sessions with anorexic patients and used those as the basis for her case histories.
16. Garner, DM, Vitousek, KM, Pike, KM, Cognitive-behavioral therapy for anorexia nervosa, Ch 7, in Garner DM, Garfinkel, PE, eds., Handbook of Treatment for Eating Disorders, second edition, New York, Guilford Press, 1997, pp. 94–144.

CHAPTER THIRTEEN

1. Hsu, LKG, Outcome of anorexia nervosa: a review of the literature (1954–1978), Arch Gen Psychiat 1980; 37:1041–1046.
2. Theander, S, Outcome and prognosis in anorexia and bulimia: some results of previous investigations, compared with those of a Swedish long-term study, J Psychiat Res 1985; 19:493–508.
3. Strober, M, Freeman, R, Morrell, W, The long-term course of severe anorexia nervosa in adolescents: survival analysis of recovery, relapse, and outcome predictors over 10–15 years in a prospective study, Int J Eat Disord 1997; 22:339–360.
4. Korndörfer, SR, Lucas, AR, Suman, VJ, Crowson, CS Krahn, LE, Melton, LJ, III, Long-term survival of patients with anorexia nervosa: a population-based study in Rochester, Minn, Mayo Clin Proc 2003; 78:278–284.
5. Hewitt PL, Coren S, Steel GD., Death from anorexia nervosa: age span and sex differences. Aging Ment Health 2001; 5:41–46.
6. National Vital Statistics Report, Center for Disease Control, 2000:50, No.15.

CHAPTER FOURTEEN

1. Killen, JD, Taylor, CB, Hammer, LD, Litt, I, Wilson, DM, Rich, T, Hayward, C, Simmonds, B, Kraemer, H, Varady, A, An attempt to modify unhealthful eating

attitudes and weight regulation practices of young adolescent girls, Int J Eating Disorders, 1993; 13:369–84.

2. Mann, T, Nolen-Hoeksema, S, Huang, K, Burgard, D Wright, A. Hanson, K, Are two interventions worse than none? Health Psychology, 1997;16:215–25.

3. Piran, N, Prevention of eating disorders: directions for future research. Psychopharmacology Bul. 1997; 33:419–23.

4. Carter, JC, Stewart, DA, Dunn, VJ, Fairburn, CG, Primary prevention of eating disorders: might it do more harm than good? Int. J. Eating Disorders 1997; 22:167–172.

5. Battle, EK, Brownell, KD, Confronting a rising tide of eating disorders and obesity treatment vs. prevention and policy, Addictive Behaviors 1996; 21:755–765.

Ginsburg, D, 38
Golden Cage, The (Bruch), 134
Göteborg, Sweden, 24
Gottllieb, Lori, 17–18
growth chart, 65
guilt, 113–114, 145
gynecologists, 92

hair, 85
Halmi, Katherine, 118
Hamer, Dean, 37, 38
Handbook of Treatment of Eating Disorders (Garner, Vitousek and Pike), 134
health, 103–104, 111
heart rate, 82
height, on growth chart, 65
history: anorexia nervosa through, 4–5; patient's diet, 125–126, 127
Hoek, HW, 23, 27
Holland, 23, 27
hormones, 81, 86, 89–90, 92
hospitalization, 15, 29–30, 106–109, 112, 116–120, 126; partial, 120–121
Hsu, George, 20, 41, 149
Huse, Diane, 125, 129
hypercarotenemia, 85
hypermetabolic conditions, 8
hyperthyroidism, 8, 80–81
hypothyroidism, 81

incidence rate, 24–26
infertility, 82. *See also* fertility
inflammatory bowel disease, 8, 77, 79–80
information, sources of, xi–xii, 3–4, 159–161
insurance, 118, 119, 120
intervention, individual, 156
ipecac, 99
It's Nobody's Fault (Koplewitz), 114

Journal of the American Dietetic Association, 129

Kalucy, RS, 24
Kaplan, AS, 121
Kendler, Kenneth, 97
ketosis, 83
Keys, Ancel, 38
Killen, JD, 154
Koplewitz, Harold, 114

laboratory tests, 9, 65, 80
laxatives, 97–98, 100–101. *See also* diarrhea
Lee, R, 92
liquids, absorption of, 84
listening, 115–116. *See also* communication
Living With Your Genes (Hamer and Copeland), 37, 38
London, England, 24, 27
Lucas, Alexander R., 21, 34–35, 53, 66, 97, 125, 129

malabsorption syndromes, 8
Mann, T, 155
marriage, 145, 147
Mayo Clinic, xiii, 33, 92, 120, 151
Mayo Clinic Diet Manual, 115, 127, 129
meal plan, 104–107, 126–129, 135, 140
meal plans, sample, 129–131
media, 3, 42, 43, 155–157
medication, 62, 98–100, 134–136. *See also* vitamins
men, bulimic disorders in, 99. *See also* gender
menstruation, 60–61, 72, 76, 81–82, 86–87, 89
mental disorders, 9–10. 16, 65–66, 70. *See also* depression
metabolic rate, 8, 40, 65, 80, 127
Meyer, Adolf, 34
Michigan Department of Mental Health, xiii
Middle East, 88
milk, 128, 135
Monroe County, New York, 21